# Caretakers
# & Lifesavers

*My Memoirs ~ To Hell and Back*

## Dale M. Bayliss

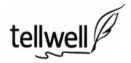

Tellwell Talent
www.tellwell.ca

ISBN
978-1-77370-025-0 (Hardcover)
978-1-77370-026-7 (Paperback)
978-1-77370-024-3 (eBook)

## Dedication

This book is dedicated to the amazing people I've had the privilege to work with throughout my long and eventful career. Every one of them is a part of me now. They are all dedicated to the cause of helping others, and they have helped me become the person I wanted to be and greatly enhanced my life, as well as my professional career. I could not have asked to be surrounded by better people.

Looking back, I consider my greatest success to be my past students, numbering over a thousand. Students whom I've had the privilege to make better, spent hours together in class, and for the rest of our careers will be able to draw on lessons learned from each other.

Finally, I want to dedicate this book to my true friends who always stood beside me throughout my career. In the worst situations, we stood our ground. When I needed you the most you were right at my side. For that I will always be grateful.

*"Sometimes we need to bend the rules to save a life, but we should not break our moral code, destroy our ethics, or lose our soul along the way."*

**Dale M. Bayliss**

# Table of Contents

# "Every Person Counts"

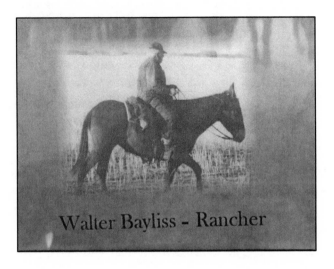

Walter Bayliss - Rancher

When I was a child I had no idea what I would be when I grew up. The small-town close to the farm I was raised on was just like any other small rural town in Saskatchewan. It had its benefits—its nice people—my relatives, neighbours, and the farming community that stuck together in times of crisis. But I had my share of personal trials and tribulations just like everyone else. I was raised eight miles (fourteen kilometres) northwest of Carnduff, Saskatchewan. Carnduff is located close to the United States and Manitoba borders. Carnduff was a great place to grow up as a child where we had miles and miles of country to explore with no real chance of being harmed. We always had unique adventures that kept us from being bored. I was considered just another farm kid by many. Everything I did as a kid made me a better person later in life, I'm sure.

I was pretty much a grown-up by the age of twelve. By then I was already working like a man and driving like an adult. Plus, if you looked at me, I was the size of an adult which is ironic considering I went from being a 3.5-pound premature twin to being the biggest and tallest student in every class. I never had to worry about working out as I already had the strength of two men, but—unfortunately— not the coordination. When it came to sports I was terrible. When it came to wearing skates or ski boots, I could never be as good as other kids were since my ankles were my kryptonite. I wore ankle supports as a kid and it helped, but not as much as I wished most days.

I have no idea how I ended up in the healthcare / EMS field. I could weld or fix almost anything, but people are more of a challenge. Yet, I always worried about people and their problems more than my own. My twin sister was always one of my first worries, and maybe it's her fault that I took on the role of being a caretaker for others in need. I bet many people are still shocked to know where I ended up. Looking back, I can truly say life is what you make it—and the more you apply or put into it, the more returns you'll get. My destiny wasn't so much predetermined as it was made with hours of hard work and dogged determination.

I only have a few regrets from my lifetime of hard work, dedication and personal commitment, and some very good lessons to share. My biggest regret is not making it all the way to the top, which to me would be an emergency room physician or a trauma doctor. But being part of the same team on many cases where lives were saved and we made a difference was close enough. Life has so many lessons to teach us that most people take for granted. I've learned the hard way over the years that life is too precious to waste even a second. Many of the lessons I am so proud of are the simple ones I learned as a kid that have taken me this far in life.

We learned how to work hard as kids, and we learned that our neighbours were also our family, and, most important, we learned that life is precious for all. I was raised on a big farm that had more animals and people around it than most. We raised horses and cows and had about forty miles of fence to fix if you ever had a boring day. I got into my share of trouble as a young teenager and we raised a little hell on the weekends but it was mostly just stuff that all country kids do.

We played hard and worked a lot harder. We had little respect for kids who had no ambition or who had no respect for our way of life or for life itself. In our world, respect was earned and friendships were permanent. We got dirt on our clothes, oil on our hands and soaked in sweat many times. We never complained and we never quit till the job was done. We had time for coffee when neighbours dropped in but then we worked until the day's work was done. I can remember in grade nine, going to school with a New Holland 1049 self-propelled bale wagon and then stacking bales until 11:00 p.m. many nights after school and having fun doing it. It was being outdoors and it was freedom like many people never know or see in a lifetime. Only a few teachers were on my side—and that made learning much harder with the majority not on my side. So, I worked harder just doing my best and staying alive doing what I had to do to get by one day at a time.

When I was sixteen years old, I was unlike most teenagers as I was already expected to help out on our farm every day. We kids had no extra time for our homework as we were needed to help my dad feed the horses, work with the cows and make sure the sheep were not being killed by predators in the winter months. During the summer, it was haying, fixing the fence, doing building repairs and anything else that we could find to do in a sixteen-hour day. My dad had a vision of what it took to be successful and self-sufficient and we were more than happy to work side by side with whomever would help with any task at hand. We could and would drive anything and were expected to help save or shoot an injured animal or rescue any animal out of a dugout or river with a rope or chain at a second's notice. Every living being was important in our world, especially our farm animals. They commonly ate before we had our lunch or supper and were looked after very well.

We were so lucky to have many dear family members close by as well. My grandma and grandpa lived just two miles east of our farm and we walked, biked or rode horses to their house often to escape reality and be treated special. Grandma was the most amazing lady in the world. Her yard was meticulous; her garden was the biggest I'd ever seen. She had the most raspberries, strawberries, and even chokecherries when the season was ready. When we needed something and Dad and Mum were away, all we had to do was make one phone call and we had support. Even if we were bad, Grandma would fix it. The funniest memory I have of my Granny Bayliss was when we used to drive past her house a little too fast. She would call and track down the driver and they would get a talking to they would not forget. Grandma would say, "You drive like hell and that is where you're going to end up" and she knew what she was talking about. Grandpa was always puttering around the yard and loved to show us stuff he had made or built. Grandpa even taught me how to weld and although I wasn't very good at it, it was my start to fixing many things that needed mending. Grandpa loved to hunt and fix stuff and I learned many things that I'll never forget from his years of wisdom. But in the end of the day Grandma was my favourite person in the whole wide world.

My Uncle Tony and Auntie Vi Day were never far away and with one call they would be right over and saved us many times. They were always just a call away. Whenever there was any kind of emergency, we could count on them. I remember one Sunday morning when

I was stacking bales in the ditches by Glen Ewan and I tipped my bale wagon onto its side while trying to stack small square bales in the steep roadside ditches. I was so scared. I thought I was dead as the bale wagon was very expensive. I wanted to call my dad but I was scared for my life even if it was not really my fault.

It wasn't my fault, though but it was the laws of physics working against me. I called Auntie Vi and told her I needed the cherry picker or a winch tractor to put my bale wagon on its wheels. I knew if I got the wagon back on its wheels I was better off and then I was praying nothing was broken. Well, let me tell you, I was so happy to see the big semi coming down the gravel road to my rescue. But right behind the cherry picker was my uncle, followed by my dad in his old farm truck. I thought for sure I'd be shot dead right there on the spot. But they all got out and had a look and said it wasn't bad at all. They hooked the cherry picker on to the bale wagon and in no time, I was back on my wheels. One little broken side rail was the only damage to the bale wagon. I took it back home and in ten minutes with a welder and a grinder it was as good as new, minus the red paint. Thank God, I was going slow when the accident happened and it was a slow roll so the damage was limited to a metal stress fracture.

There were not very many tasks or chores that we did not do and when they were completed my dad could always find us more work. I was somewhat mechanically inclined but not as much as my brother, Donnie. My other two brothers had their unique skills, as well. My brother Russel was a farmer and a rancher from the time he was a little kid. I was never into working with animals or chasing or herding cows or horses, as I wanted to spend my spare time working on the broken machinery.

I would rather be working on tractors than working with livestock, so I got to do jobs that where intended for drivers instead of riders. I could ride a horse, but it wasn't my first choice of transportation.

I had no idea then that I would soon leave the farm and take up a new occupation that was little known to others in my community. I would soon be doing a job most people I knew would hate or would flat-out never want to do or attempt.

One hot summer day, I was stacking bales with our self-propelled bale wagon for a local rancher / farmer close to Alameda, Saskatchewan, when, little did I know, my life would change direction. While listening to our local radio station I heard the announcer talking about a fatal accident between a truck and a bicycle north of Carnduff, my home town. I was shocked when I heard that the person killed was Jamie Stevenson. Jamie was a well-respected kid in our little town with a sister in my class, who I always thought was very nice, as well as a little brother and a great set of parents. Jamie was one of the good guys.

Jamie's dad worked at the local New Holland store and his mother worked at the local post office. Jamie was one of the few town kids that would give me the time of day and not be a snob to me or my family when our paths crossed. Jamie was always happy to see me and meant something to me. I knew he would always be there if I needed to talk and was someone to count on in times of trouble.

A truck accidentally struck Jamie while he was riding his bike by a half-ton truck on a very poor, narrow highway straight north of town. Jamie lay there and slowly died of his internal injuries and no one came to his rescue. The fact that there were no ambulances in our community and no ambulances available for sixty miles that day made it so he had no chance to live. Jamie's death was an unfortunate event and his life could likely have been saved in today's system, but unfortunately not back then. Jamie died due to a system that did not seem to care about sick or injured patients as it was not an established medical system at that time. There were also frequent industrial accidents that occurred within the nearby oil industry that needed medical attention but would rarely get it in time.

There was no service in the area for the local farmers, ranchers, labourers or retired residents throughout our small communities who were not aware that EMS could help them in times of need if it was available. This was partially due to the fact that the majority of taxpayers and councilors in our surrounding communities had no idea of the true need for modern emergency medical services. They did not realize that lives could be helped and suffering could be lessened if they had modern basic life support BLS services, which provide a higher level of care then what was available at the current time. Just prior to the current BLS services, almost all ambulances were run from the local funeral homes. They provided a great service as a scoop-and-run but, elsewhere, EMS was evolving.

I later heard that Jamie was alive for some time on scene, but for multiple reasons he just lay on the highway and died a slow death. It was no one's fault but, regardless, there was no immediate aid. There was no local ambulance and there were no trained emergency medical responders even close to our town or in our municipality. I was angry that there was no one who could help the injured or the sick when they needed it most. There were many people who got injured or had a medical emergency who would collapse and die long before help arrived. They had no hope to live long enough to see their dreams be fulfilled. I knew that not everyone could or would be saved even with the best medical care, but I wanted to at least give them an opportunity. I thought if we could even save or help 10 per cent of the people who could not help themselves that would be one hell of a start. We could make a difference for many who deserved a chance to live a better life. People didn't have to die from certain injures if the right medically trained people could come and help them in times of need.

After that day, there was a strange desire in my heart to change my sometimes-uncaring attitude and try to help others. I do not think I was full of hate or spite, but as a teenager you do not normally think of helping others before yourself or being in the medical industry as a teenager I'm sure. The role of an EMS modern responder was slowly expanding and I could see potential in the role of the EMTs. I knew the role of the EMT could make the difference in many others especially in our local community.

I knew right then that someone had to be able to help the injured or sick in our communities at a local level at any time, anywhere, and at anyplace. I had no idea of the challenges I would face or the numbers of tragedies I would come across but I was determined and was not going to look the other way. If people needed help when they were sick or hurt I would learn what I needed to and they would be helped. They would not lay and die without someone helping them; if I could help them, I would be there 24/7. If I had to work twenty-four hours a day and seven days a week, I would do it.

I had already witnessed a few relatives and one other friend die tragically and thought with a little bit of training there had to be something I could do if I had the guts and the heart to be an Emergency Medical Responder (EMR). Just my family alone could have used an ambulance at least ten times I'm sure, and how many other times would there be a need with our neighbours and friends? During that time, I liked TV shows that were medically related in any way. I also liked any show having anything to do with police and fire services. Even if it was just a cartoon; it was worth watching or reading.

I was sure that even just one person at the right time in a rapid response vehicle could come to the scene and they would make the difference even with simple interventions of the airway, breathing, and oxygen therapy. One thing we took for granted for too long was the importance to stopping bleeding thus decreasing the effects of shock. We just needed to get to the scene fast enough. The more we learned the more we could help people as we were able to expand our scope of practice.

I somehow knew even back then that if someone was meant to die they would, regardless of their injuries or illness. But later in life I also learned that we could save a lot more if we just gave 110 per cent every day on every patient. We could and would change destiny of many with the effort of the trained few. If we could apply some lifesaving interventions early we could prevent the pending cardiac or respiratory arrest. As we learn more and more we learn the cause of the illness or the effects of the injury need to be addressed early to change the outcomes.

I thought about where I could make the most difference in others' lives and concluded that it would be in the Emergency Medical Services (EMS) at a very young age. I needed a purpose that I could see me doing for the rest of my life and it was not being a farmer or a rancher. The only way I thought that I could make a difference was to become a paramedic. I just needed a way to get there, and a little bit of luck along the way wouldn't hurt.

Many times, in my life, I would hit a brick wall, but it never stopped me. I got over the wall, even if it sometimes left me emotionally hurt or scared. I would take the hit and go onto the next person in need and then to the next as soon as possible. In the amazing movie, "The Guardian", Kevin Costner's character - Ben Randall, tells hotshot - Jake Fisher, "Save the ones you can, Jake. The rest, you've got to let them go." I would not see this movie until it came out in 2006. After it came out, I must have watched it at least ten times. Many of the parts about Ben as a US Coast Guard aviation survival technician at the end of a really good career were similar to my own life experiences. The consequences of spending your life helping others are not all good. We can do our best for years but it comes at a cost to us physically, mentally and emotionally.

It's so true that what doesn't kill us makes us stronger, but also every interaction we have with our surroundings changes our destiny. It also changes our patients' and their family's destinies in ways we may never be able to measure. When you are dedicated to giving 110 per cent to every patient, the outcomes are improved but at a hidden cost. Many times, I would assume someone's pain and take over their situation and make it better in any way possible at any cost. I never settled for just doing enough when I could do even more. Even if it meant my shift was longer and my sleep shorter, it was worth it every time. If someone needed help they would get it, whether it was medical, mechanical or an errand; we made their world better.

All in all, it was worth the heartbreak and the tears I shed trying to make things better even when it was a losing battle. I saw so many patients who would not have made it without us all fighting for their life. Sometimes we were fighting a system of chaos and we made the right decisions for the best available outcome possible. At the end of the day we would all do our best for the patients and their families.

I had no idea that the average paramedic from the late 1970s was so under-educated, under-recognized, and underpaid. Over the next thirty-five years I had no idea of the personal hardships I would face that would be both mentally challenging and physically draining. Nor did I have a true sense of the tragedies that would cross my path and the rewards that I would receive. The majority of rewards came from the satisfaction I got from doing the right thing. These rewards were very personal as they came from the hearts of the patients that I had the privilege to help. I helped them with their personal battles or struggles to live and stay alive and every one of them mattered to me, regardless of why they needed help.

I also learned over the years that giving too much was not necessarily the best idea, but after being used to always giving 110 percent to everyone it caused me pain watching others only give 70 or 90 percent effort. It was, and still is, hard to watch fellow colleagues look the other way when others need help. When I witnessed patients being treated poorly, I would always step in, even if it made people mad at me. I knew I would have to push myself to my limits to make a difference in the profession.

Over time I built an inner strength from personal wisdom and a desire to be the best I could be, all while trying to be humble, caring and compassionate to those in need. I always tried to give everyone the benefit of the doubt, but if you crossed the line I was done. I had a rule that if it was going to turn out bad, I had to win at any cost to me. I would not let people hit me when I was down. I would never just stand there and watch others hurt anyone else, ever. I would also never let my coworkers or partners get hurt or pushed around, even by other colleagues.

Many times, I ended up getting stitches, scars, or bruises, as well as being disciplined verbally, for coming to someone's aid, but it was fine with me. I could not look the other way or change that about myself even if it killed me. Often, when people got into trouble or were threatened at work, they would call me and several of my good friends and I would go and try to help in any way we could. Often, I was in the right place at the wrong time and got hit or knocked over. Sometimes the presence of extra staff would deter someone who was trying to intimidate or physically hurt other staff members. No matter the pain, the suffering or complications I would endure, I would not let others down or allow them to suffer in times of need. If I said I was your friend, I was your friend. If you had my number, I was only a call away.

Over the years, I even backed up the RCMP a few times and helped save the life of someone who needed non-medical assistance in the worst way. When I came running over and helped perform a careful takedown or a skilled tackle, they were very thankful on every occasion. I never thought about my own safety on these occasions, as it was just who I was and I knew someone needed help. I would not look the other way if someone needed help.

I used to think and told a few good friends that we were "care-takers and heartbreakers," as we always tried our best, but would sometimes end up breaking the hearts of the patient's loved ones, regardless. I would not let a student, or a partner, only do enough for a patient if they needed more than the care that was given. Over the years, I have made many personal mistakes in my life. My decisions have made my life more challenging than it probably needed to be, but it has made me who I am today. Learning from our mistakes is essential. I believe it is why I have grown into who I am today. So, in the end, I can't have many regrets about my life, as I only can change the future. Thankfully, life can offer us insight into our past and show us more about who we are through paying attention to the lessons it teaches us.

In this book, I talk about my successes as well as my failures. Many of these failures have been great learning opportunities for me that I have shared with my students and coworkers. If we could all go back in time and change one thing, I would do so in a heartbeat, but I know things sometimes happen for a purpose we may never truly comprehend or understand. Sometimes we end up doing the wrong thing for the right reasons and sometimes we end up doing the right thing for the wrong reasons.

In the end, we must all live with our decisions and, better yet, we need to be able to sleep with them. This is the part that isn't always easy. We all strive to do our best in the world of helping others and saving lives, but the rules are not all black and white. There are some areas that are "crystal clear," but many others that are grey or completely unknown. Life is meant to be lived forward and retrospective reflection is nice but it's only a small part of our conscious thought. Living is an unconscious act, and we often rely on our instinctual physiological response—our "fight or flight response"—when we are personally challenged or physically threatened. This is more common in stressful situations than most people can understand. As first responders, we always do what we know best in times of stress and the more prepared we are, the more options we can come up with under duress. That is why we need to train hard to always make the best decisions possible under such serious conditions.

My most humbling experience has been helping my students to be better people than before our paths crossed. I would tell them of my life experiences and share with them my personal mistakes when I could to prevent them from making the same ones.

We all make mistakes sometimes. It's the question of "At what cost to the patient?" that I would always ask myself. Sometimes we need to fail to learn, and learning comes from our making decisions that are not always the best. Over time we all learn or should learn from our mistakes.

I know my pain, the suffering and the loneliness, would always be worth the time out of my life to make it right for others. This lyric from Matt Anderson's song, "When My Angel Gets the Blues," says it all for me: "Little girl, I'll follow you down, I don't care how far we go, I need to see you get your feet back on the ground. You don't need to tell me, 'cause I don't need to know." Sometimes we don't need to know the reasons others are hurt or down on life but we need to bring them back safe. No matter what it takes, it is what we must do. If we need to rescue a lost friend, we go and get them or bring them back. If we see people in distress, we help them when we can. The more we know our friends, the more we may need to put ourselves out there and help them when life gets tough.

In this book, I will try to show you how my life unfolds with the good and bad times. As we get older we keep learning, and as we learn we also change from within. Life is too precious to waste. Regardless of our race, colour or personal beliefs, we are all required to live and function together. Personally, I wish we could have kept closer as a family and worked out our unique problems to help each other even more than we did in the past.

I hope you enjoy reading about the experiences that taught me the best lifelong lessons. May your heart and your life be touched by my stories of helping others while, at the same time, I was going through some good but also some very bad times in my life. Overall, I can say my career has been very rewarding and I have many good memories from while I was on the job. My ultimate dream would be that others carry on my desire to "pay it forward" to anyone in need. I would love to build Dale's Foundation to Care so more people around the globe can benefit from the efforts of first responders.

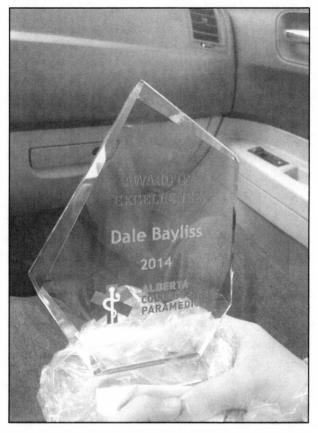

*Award of Excellence 2014 "Everyone Counts"*

# "We All Need a Reason"

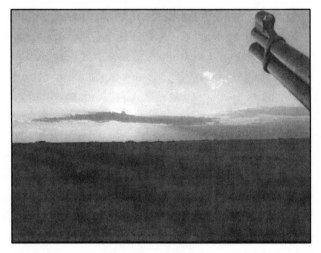

*"A Reason"*

My first introduction to the EMS world was by taking first aid and CPR courses, which were offered by the American Red Cross from an American instructor. This was truly amazing. We didn't have a local instructor at that time within sixty miles, I'm sure. The US had CPR available from the American Red Cross before Canada even considered it and we ended up crossing the border for the initial CPR course. That was when it was so easy to enter the US or come back across and no passports or identification were needed at all. What stood out the most to me about the coursework was the speed at which EMS arrived on the scene and the level of contact first responders had when it came to the patient. You got the call and you got to work. Patients needed rescue breathing, or mouth-to-mouth ventilation which was the only way before the pocket mask or barrier devices became standard. Or they needed chest compressions, which are the most important part of CPR. But if they were alive, the active bleeding was the next most important concern to address and this was such a practical approach.

During my early days of training, I had very little knowledge into the pathophysiology, the cellular interactions and the delicate balance it takes to keep people out of system failure. The most important lesson that anyone needs to know is that the human body may display general signs and symptoms of complications, but unless we fix the cellular event that initiated the problem everything fails. I quickly learned the importance of the heart and lungs and how they interact uniquely, as we often attended to patients in arrest due to cardiorespiratory failure or cardiorespiratory collapse. In the early days, I had no idea the delicate effects trauma had on infants and the elderly, or the effects of diabetes on the heart or the circulatory system, along with the effects of the golden hour on comorbidity factors. Over time I would learn that children younger than five years old can die from trauma or burns all too easily, and that those over sixty can die from even minor trauma.

Sometime in the fall of 1981, I enrolled in the Emergency Medical Technician course in Carnduff, Saskatchewan, at the age of just sixteen years old. The course was part-time in Carnduff and part-time in Estevan, Saskatchewan. When I enrolled in the EMT course, I did not tell them I was only sixteen years old and they never asked. It wasn't until after I was in the course for a little while that someone figured it out. On my first exam, I had no idea of what to expect and I scored a low 63 percent. I wasn't prepared for the level of difficulty or the types of questions that would be asked. I then thought about what I needed to do to get a better mark and I never had a mark of less than 90 percent after that day with a final average of 89 percent in the course.

The only problem was that I had failed my practical scenarios and I had to then redo the complete course. They won if that was their job for they had failed me, but I wasn't done yet. I would not quit and swore that day to make it up the EMS hill or die trying. I wanted to be mentored in the industry and when your leader is great, so will you be in time. I just had to do what was needed to make it. I wasn't prepared for the type of scenarios I was presented with and had no idea how to handle the scenario games. I would face the scenario games over the next number of years of trying to be an EMT and eventually a paramedic, and I won, but not easily. In the end, I would master the scenario games and helped ensure that my students made it up and over the same hurdles I'd faced.

During the first Emergency Medical Technician – Ambulance (EMT-A) course, I had the opportunity to do a ride along with Supreme Ambulance Care in Carlyle. Supreme Ambulance Care had a very busy service with a high call volume. They had amazing units and state-of-the-art equipment. The service looked after everyone from the few small towns and surrounding municipalities. They also serviced a local First Nations reserve which had its share of issues stemming from violence and self-destructiveness. Many of the community members were affected by the introduction of their community to different kinds of alcohol and drugs, which, sadly, also included prescription medications and not just illegal drugs.

Many seniors, kids and even infants on the reserve were affected directly or indirectly from family members doing drugs or by abusing alcohol. Pain causes so much physical, mental and emotional complications for so many people in this world.

The origins of this pain are not even that hard to see or understand if you take the time to look into the effects of alcohol on Indigenous cultures. So much of this tragedy stems from the lack of ability to break down alcohol at a cellular level in Indigenous populations compared to, for example, Europeans, who have been drinking alcohol for more than 5000 years. Alcohol had only been introduced to North American Indigenous people some 300 years ago. Alcohol has such different effects on all races, and not just Indigenous people. It can have harmful effects on the very young and the elderly, and patients with kidney or liver disease are also affected negatively.

After riding in a few ambulances, I could see Supreme Ambulance Care was one of the leaders in EMS care in our area. I knew from the look of the excellent equipment and the quality of the members. They had pride in their work and were dedicated to helping others despite cultural or ethnic differences. They had pride in the EMS care they provided but, more important, they showed pride in what they did for others. This is most likely one of the most important aspects needed for an EMT to be an effective member of a health care team. With pride, there is improved teamwork, and patients have the best chance to do better in the long run. With a team, you can take the worst-case scenario and make some good come out of it.

The local owner-operator of Supreme Ambulance Care was also assisting in teaching our local EMT-A course in Carnduff and Estevan. I admired Lou's experience but he also had a side that was not so nice to me and the other students, but at the time it was not clear to me why. I wonder, looking back, if he was just trying to scare us or, more likely, he was probably suffering from PTSD as well as compassion fatigue. There is no way you can do what he did and not be affected. I wish I could have learned more from him in the time we had together.

From his stories, I'm sure Lou was affected by the same events that break many people—even the toughest ones break and the scars run deep. No one can come face-to-face with tragedy over and over and not be affected. Many of the events that you see as an EMT cannot be shared with very many people. You also can't block them from your memory easily. I seriously think Lou wanted to make sure we had the guts and the heart to do the job right. We had to earn our right to make it our passion or lifelong mission, even though it might secretly not have been his lifelong dream. I will never know the answer but I've sure thought about it a lot. I just wish I could sit down with Lou now and ask him that one question. I think I would see a completely different person. I would love to be his partner today, even if he still intimated me.

I know Lou would have made a great paramedic if he was given the chance. It must have been hard for him trying to help others who were so messed up for so many sad reasons, knowing he could have done more if he had the training and the opportunity. Sometimes the pure helplessness breaks us apart more than others will ever know. Lou essentially said that we should get out while we can if we didn't have the guts to continue. I have never forgotten Lou and I respect him greatly for his little lessons as they were not always textbook lessons but good lifelong lessons that don't fit in any medical textbook. Lou, I'm here today to show you I had the guts. I also had the determination even if I never dreamed of the hardship the job would cost my inner soul from time to time. The challenges and the changes to me from within would make my life better for the reason that they have made me who I am today. I work very hard and ensure I provide the extra care needed to help anyone in need. Lou, I made it in spite of everyone who tried to stop me along the way. Thanks for pushing me ahead and, in the end, you made me a better EMT, so our paths crossing was never a negative event.

I realized that if I was going to be in the EMS industry, I would have to prove myself by going that extra mile for the people who did not have the strength or ability to go on. Taking the EMT course again did not deter me but increased my knowledge and dedication. I knew what I wanted and I would not be deterred in my plans to help people, as it was my only real dream and dreams are what make miracles happen. Dreams are realized through dedication and persistence.

I initially worked in Grenfell, Saskatchewan, as my first real EMS job for about a month was for a BLS ambulance service. I had no idea back then of what was needed to be an EMT, from stethoscopes to uniforms which most employers did not supply. It was a good service but I didn't see eye-to-eye with the manager and I knew it was no place to start my career. I was so young and naive at that time and being only sixteen years old, I had no idea what to expect. I remember Peter and Wendy who took me under their wing and gave me enough education, or simple wisdom, about EMS to get started. They showed me professionalism that I had no idea even existed in EMS. Peter was a great EMT but you could tell his dream was to be a police officer someday. I hope Peter made it into the RCMP, as that was one of his wishes way back then and he looked like a police officer already. Peter had the right mentality for being an officer of the law. It's just too bad I never got to see them again and we lost contact.

I remember several calls from back then, but two of them come to mind as educational calls. I do have a memory of a single vehicle rollover where a young girl and her brother from Cartwright, Manitoba, had rolled their truck. Apparently, a passing motorist, whom I believe was an off-duty RCMP member, lifted the back end of the vehicle off her prior to our arrival and very likely saved her life. I found the call to be a reality check that our patients are very much human and we need to go that extra mile to help them. They need to know we are there to help them make it through their time of crisis. It was one of the few times I felt extremely nauseated after the call and I'm still not sure to this day why it only hit me after the call, in the hospital. Also, looking back, it goes to show us that when the right person is present in the right place at the right time, it makes all the difference. That was one of the many monumental calls during my career.

I thought I had learned all I could in my EMT course and I had a fairly good idea of what medical terminology was all about until that 3:00 a.m. call from a patient who called our emergency line and requested an ambulance. He stated, "I'm a hemophiliac and I fell down tonight and I need my Factor VIII." I thought he was crazy and I think my partners did, as well. On arrival, we found a nice but intoxicated male who had fallen after drinking a little too much alcohol and needed to go to the hospital for a Factor VIII infusion. I soon realized there might be a few other books that I might need to read in the near future if I was going to master the bleeding disorder complications.

I started working EMS and vowed to take the EMT course ASAP—I would show them all this was my life and my future! In the winter of 1983, I was old enough to get into the next EMT course and it would be my next step in my EMS career. While I was taking the course, I was sitting in the front lobby of St. Joseph Hospital in Estevan on a practical skills day. I was just sitting in the hospital waiting room waiting for class to start and killing time, reading. Suddenly a car pulled up in front of the emergency entrance. A bystander apparently came across the accident and brought this broken kid directly to the hospital. A crew was already out looking for him but the bystander beat them all and transported him by car.

He was clearly hurt very badly but still walked into the hospital on his own, even with his face smashed in. I helped guide him to the emergency room and we all yelled for help. I couldn't get him to follow commands, so I just picked him up and laid him on the stretcher and the doctors, nurses and staff went to work on him right away. Later that day I heard he actually inhaled a tooth into his lungs and died from head trauma in addition to other complications. If anyone could have done more it would have been done, I'm positive.

It was a rural hospital doing the best they could do and there was no one to blame but the three-wheel ATV and the travelling conditions that created the accident. Later on, three-wheel ATVs would be banned because of calls like this and the tragedy they left in their wake. After 1987, it was made illegal to then sell three-wheel ATVs. By 1988, it was illegal to manufacture them at all as they were deemed unsafe. I wonder how many people they killed in such a short time frame. The thought of the number of parents who lost kids due to ATV accidents over my lifespan is heartbreaking.

Looking at it now from the perspective of our current education and training, I'm sure we could have handled this patient so much differently. With the right trained people and the right medications to lessen the severe head injury and side effects, maybe he could have stood a chance. But this was before CT scanners were commonplace, and before we understood the true meaning of mean arterial pressure (MAP), or the effects on the brain from increased intracranial pressure (ICP) from closed head injuries. Everything changed with the introduction of the Monro-Kellie doctrine. Basically, this hypothesis states that the space in the cranium is limited and any type of bleeding, swelling or extra lesion takes up valuable space. Regardless, the aspiration pneumonia in this case was not something that could easily be fixed, and it would have taken an expert to remove the tooth from the boy's lung.

Over time, I learned that some people would do better and others would do worse with certain head injuries. Ironically, it seemed only alcoholics could get away with the acute and chronic bleeds they would get from falling so often. Seeing as they had a shrunken brain already, they could tolerate a little more bleeding. They just needed to be monitored by neurosurgical services closely and if they decompensated they were off to the operating room (OR) for life-saving surgery. The healthy eighteen to thirty-year-olds were usually not so lucky, as their brains were at their biggest and functioning at their prime. So, it was always wise to consider age and past medical history with all patients. If only they had trained trauma teams in those days, there could have been more lives saved. We all had so much to learn, but medical education was much more limited than it is today.

When it came time for me to take the EMT course, I was more than ready. I just wanted to be an emergency medical technician – ambulance attendant. The EMT course was being offered in Oxbow and Estevan, with a Practicum in Regina which really opened my eyes and gave me a purpose in life. The biggest problem was I needed more and more practice and had no one on my side to make the next step. From the time, I started the EMT Course and throughout I found a desire to be the best of the best. I started as about the last and ended up with the higher marks. I just needed practical experience and someone who believed in me. I also really needed a mentor in my life. I know what it is like being on a losing team and trying to be a winner if you're going at it alone. This was a familiar story I'd seen many times in my life and knowing that I wasn't going to ever quit. Failure wasn't an option as I'd rather die trying then quit. The only quote from my English class came right from *Julius Caesar:* "A coward dies a thousand times before his death, but the valiant never taste of death but once." Quitting wasn't an option. I knew I could make it if I worked hard and kept trying. Someday I'd make it out of the park. Someday I'd hit a home run. I knew it could happen. Then one day when I wasn't even thinking about it, it just happened.

I graduated from the EMT course and now I could finally work as an EMT. I wanted to work in my home town or in the immediate area. I knew people in my area needed me as they were always short of EMTs for our local ambulances services. Over the next thirty years I'd see many different types of providers—some were very good and were true professionals and others not so much. Some were there in uniform but that was about it. We would also see and work out of many different types of ambulances over the years that all had unique challenges. Later, I would get to work out of planes and helicopters, as well. More important, I was privileged to work with some dedicated, brilliant and caring individuals who now make up my EMS family. Over time you realize that with the right people, the right equipment, being in the right place at the right time, as well as having the right transport, you actually can make saving lives or helping others easy. If everything lines up, our job can be easy and if fate or destiny is against us, the day will be hell.

Transportation of our patients is sometimes overrated. As long as you get there in one piece, you're good. If we can get to the patient in enough time to abort the internal chaos, we can alter destiny in the majority of cases. We can alleviate suffering, help stabilize the sick or the injured, and we save as many lives as possible. But sometimes a patient's fate has already been decided and it isn't in the cards that they should live. We can't defeat death when we aren't meant to win, but we will sure as hell try. I remember fighting my whole shift for patients and losing in the end, anyway. But on other occasions, we won. Sometimes you need to count the wins in life and not the losses. The best lesson I can give you in this chapter is to save the ones you can and then carry on, even if your heart is broken you must keep going ahead in life. We all lose some battles, the hardest fight to save a life but we help and save many of our very sick patients. I wonder just maybe somedays heaven needs more angels, so every once in a while, we need to admit defeat and just know it was meant to be even if we don't know the why or the bigger reason.

Over time, I learned that if I could alleviate pain, decrease suffering and provide comfort to the victim's family in emergency situations, I had mastered my role as an EMT. Sometimes holding someone's hand tightly or letting them die with dignity matters more than anything else. Dying alone or letting people die in pain is never right. We are there to help our patients and their families through the worst times in their life. The pain we witness on a daily basis is not something that is easy to share.

Throughout our life, we lose little bits of our soul on bad days, but with time we do heal. We might never be the same as when we started, but we go on. At the end of the day we are always a team and must come back as a team. When we lose someone, it affects us all and our overall team is therefore changed. The dynamics of every team is always different. Some teams can take on anything and make something good come out of every situation. With the right leadership from the right person, the team will ultimately overcome every obstacle they face. The outcome will be the best it could be in spite of the circumstances involved.

Saving lives is an art, and your ability to practice your art is only as good as your team. You're also only as good as the equipment you have on your call or in your emergency room. With the right medications and the wisdom to know when to use them, you can change the outcomes in many situations. You just need to know when certain medications are needed or when to use your advanced life support skills. Also, knowing when a situation demands an expert and when it's best to leave the situation alone and seek a higher level of care is very important. As a first responder, you get many quiet hours to reflect on the more complex calls and you begin to understand some of the issues that were unique about the situations. On rare occasions, the experts will stop and educate you on the next steps that would either help or hinder your patient's outcomes.

One of the most valuable initial lessons I learned in my early days in the EMS field was that you can't take life too seriously. You must deal with life as it comes to you. Decide on a pathway and live with the consequences. Over time, you will see how your decisions affect others and down the road, you can make more informed decisions. You have to care about your life, care about others, learn and customize your life to meet the challenges you come across along the way. Lauren MacRae, whose house I lived at for the last one-and-a-half years of my nursing training, put me in my place one time, letting me know "I don't care" wasn't the wisest answer and telling me I had better come up with something else. Lauren was a nurse and a second-year instructor at SIAST, though I never had her as a teacher. But the lessons she and her husband, Dr. Don MacRae, taught me during the time I lived with them will stay with me forever.

I cannot and will not ever forget the support I got from the MacRaes and the difference they made in my life. They were superb role models. The lessons I learned from them and from just living my life made me a better person. These lessons would be worth the cost of working in a stressful environment that caused me a lot of pain. There will always be someone who makes you take stock of your life and realize that you matter and that your life has purpose. My overall goal in life is to just make a difference and help one person at a time and then go on to the next one. I will always be thankful to the people who helped me on my journey. I'm just trying to pay it forward to the thousands of people who just need a little help along the way. The rewards are worth the pain and the pain is always a sign that shows you still care enough to keep playing the game of life.

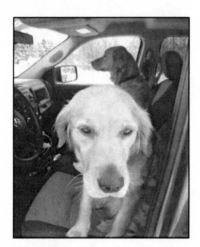

*"My reasons to live on a really bad day."*

*Chapter 2: An Introduction to the EMS Life*

# "What Does It Really Take?"

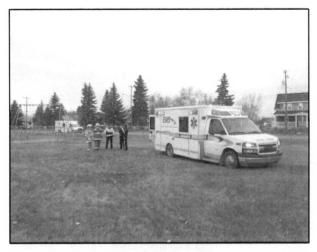

*"EMS the Right Way"*

I started my real ambulance career in Oxbow, Saskatchewan, as a casual ambulance attendant to replace the local EMT attendants when they needed a day off. In the olden days, they had one EMT and one person as a driver on every call. It was a great start and I worked casually and then full-time in Oxbow, with the odd shift in Carnduff until March of 1984, when I was hired as the co-manager along with Allen Needham, EMT-A. I did not have my EMT certificate yet and Allen was registered and willing to work part-time with me when he was not farming. Allen was the only other EMT in town at that time and was a very dedicated individual who possessed wisdom beyond his years. We did many calls together over the first year in Oxbow. Allen was in my initial EMT class and he was my relief when I needed a day off.

I soon found out what it was like to work twenty-nine days of the month and not get paid very much. We had pagers that were not reliable and only worked on their own schedule. Most of the time we relied on the phones at home or at work for that reason. We were expected to be on call 24/7 for all but a few days every month. We had to pay for our own uniforms and our education. The salary was not very high but it was someplace to start and it was all I needed at the time. It didn't pay all the bills so I needed to work two jobs just to survive. Regardless, I made it work. Eventually, my wages went up so that I was earning about $1100.00 a month. When our pagers became unreliable, I even bought a new hand-held radio for $1100 dollars so the hospital could find me when I was needed.

I worked a few casual shifts with the Carnduff Borderline Ambulance, which was a Basic Life Support (BLS) ambulance, but it was different from the Oxbow & Area Road Ambulance Service for several reasons. For one thing, there wasn't a hospital in Carnduff. Plus, they serviced a bigger area and had less equipment to work with. They also had a really small engine (no power at all) in a big van, which never was a good idea for an emergency unit. Overall, I enjoyed the work much better in Oxbow as we had a hospital to work out of and it was a little bit busier, plus we had extra equipment at our disposal. There was a little more co-operation with the hospital and the ambulance board, which meant they were making progress in the EMS world and not staying stagnant.

In those early days, we had a "gutless" ambulance, which couldn't do much more than the speed limit on a good day with a strong headwind. We also had an older Ferno Model 28 one-man stretcher, which was very common back in those days. The one-man stretcher was also commonly used by the local undertakers and was just easier to use then the first Ferno two-man stretchers. Its major drawback was it wasn't ideal for larger patients and for sure not big enough for bariatric patients. Anyone over 350 pounds and it would have been a lost cause for everyone involved. The old stretcher offered less lifting, which was nice but not as practical as our modern stretchers. To this day, the one-man stretchers are still used for body removals. Today we have completely electric and bariatric stretchers that make us feel almost archaic if we worked twenty or thirty years ago.

In those days, there was such a thing as a one-person ambulance. I never did an ambulance call by myself when I started EMS, but a few years sooner and I would have I'm sure. Although, looking back, I asked my brother to come with me one day as we had no one that would answer the phone for a rodeo accident. So, it was him or no one and off we went. On arrival, we found a nice cowgirl, with an obvious broken leg, in agony, and we went to work. My brother got promoted to being the driver after we got her into the unit. A quick check of vital signs and we were off to the local hospital, knowing her day was far from over. Elevation and ice around the splint was our BLS approach to good care. Back then we had Entonox but seldom used it. Looking back, we could and should have used it more. It's amazing how wisdom makes you change your practices for the right reasons, which are always the patient. The term "scoop and run" was exactly what it sounded like. You grabbed your patient and make a mad dash for the local emergency room. That day we just scooped and ran.

The Emergency Medical Technician course back in the day was good, but limited. The simple truth is that people were doing their best with what they had learned from past tragic experiences. You essentially learned what to do from seeing or managing a bad event in the past. It was also helpful if you were mechanically inclined, as you could figure out how to extricate patients when it came to farming accidents or mangled vehicles.

In the early days, we did our best but didn't really know how to be methodical and efficient in our actions. The EMT course was a great introduction to EMS but lacked the step-by-step format needed to put it all together. It was almost like building a jigsaw puzzle without seeing the big picture. We didn't know anything about the newest Basic Trauma Life Support course (BTLS), which was only available in the United States at the time. We had some very good practitioners doing their best and it was better than nothing, but at times not good enough. When I moved to Alberta in the summer of 1989, they had already incorporated the BTLS concepts ahead of most other provinces. This one course made a difference in so many lives. I got it under my belt as soon as it became available in Canada. When I look back to what was done in the pre-hospital care setting in Saskatchewan during the start of my career in the early 1980s, I realize that it was the most basic or lowest level of care in the EMS industry. Still, we did our best despite the lack of good training.

What we could do was basically insert an oral pharyngeal airway (OPA) to open a patient's airway and start CPR if needed, then drive like hell to the local hospital just so the on-call physician could tell us what we already knew: "Sorry your patient is still just as dead." We could not do enough for so many patients. Many just needed simple defibrillation, intravenous (IV) therapy or IV fluid boluses, simple interventions that today, even EMTs can perform. We did not see a bag-valve-mask (BVM) until about 1985 in our ambulance, which is the hallmark of artificial ventilation used to provide ventilation to any patient who is in respiratory distress, cardiac arrest or has a low breathing rate commonly known as hypoventilation. We had no idea of the unique benefit or harm oxygen might cause for another twenty years. Our doctors were not trained in using pharmacology to restart the heart, as was beginning to be a trend in many urban locations. We did our best and prayed we could be fast enough in many cases. We fought like crazy to get our patients to a higher level of care, knowing all too often that it was already too late. But we tried anyway. It was all we could do.

Looking back to what we had to deal with, I don't know how we did it. Compared to what we have today and the change in the equipment and the resources is unbelievable. It took more than just education to work EMS even when I started. It took dedication to be able to help people. You needed to actually like your job to care and you needed to always be ready to change your plans and make the best out of every minute of every day. You would make plans and they would change as suddenly as the pager went off or your phone rang. In no time, you were speeding towards the hospital, grabbing your unit, all while making sure you had a partner. Then you both had to figure out where you were going and, most important, what was awaiting you on your arrival, if known at all.

On arrival, you were the director of someone else's bad day and it was always a different patient, a unique event—no two patients have the same complications or history of preceding events. We got to learn that the mechanism of injury (MOI) was a very good predictor if your day was going to get better after being dispatched or if it was going to get worse. Sometimes the dispatch information was good, but it often didn't add up to what you found on scene. So many times, the story was unknown or the events were so unrealistic you wondered how the hell that could have happened, but it did. Over the years, you learned some things aren't in any EMS or medical textbook and somedays things just happen. You learned that you needed the dispatch information as soon as possible, then considered the MOI and then decided what you would needed to do on arrival. You also knew if fire should be dispatched or you needed a tow truck to help with the rescue.

We quickly learned about the golden hour, which was the crucial time between the time of the accident and the patient's arrival at the hospital. The first ten minutes of the golden hour were very important. It was your goal to spend the shortest time on scene possible to increase your patient's chances of survival. We only had a few options for good hospitals with sick patients and if you were a BLS provider, it wasn't good, as it would be thirty to forty minutes' transport time on a good day to a hospital with a surgeon or a blood bank. We almost always had to stop at the local hospital and stabilize first and then make another mad dash for the next hospital. With most sick patients, we were very good at loading and transporting them quickly. The problem was if you couldn't get them out of the house for any number of reasons, including size, safety or structural issues. Then you were in trouble.

Looking back to how much we learned from then to now, we could see there was a huge assessment and treatment change that could improve our overall patient care. A great example of the need to change our practice comes from the recent research in the US regarding the use of a simple blood test. If we were able to perform a serum lactate level test, we could help our geriatric patients in trauma cases. If the results of the test are over 2.0 mmol/L, it is a good predictor of serious geriatric trauma. It's amazing that a simple blood draw can give us a person's current lactate level.

We have not even realized this in Canada yet, but it will come in a few years, I hope, for the sake of our senior population. It takes more time to effect change than it should in such a modern world. I have often seen a five to ten-year delay in health care trends to cross over from the USA to the Canadian health care system. I recognize that Canada has many unique challenges, and practices are not the same from province to province. We are one but really, we aren't, as standards of health care vary widely between the provinces and territories and are also different in urban and rural settings.

Starting out, we often worked very long days. I can remember driving until you couldn't see or stay awake and switching with your partner. Then your partner would drive until the need to close their eyes was more than yours and you would take over again. We also had our regular day jobs and this was often challenging and difficult as you never knew when you would get an EMS call, and you could be gone for a few hours or for the rest of the day. I was fortunate in my first job to work at the local Massey Ferguson dealership where they gave me the opportunity to come and go on emergencies. Len, who was the shop manager, was the old ambulance owner and he always stuck up for me. Len knew what our worst days were like for he had walked many more miles then i had in my EMS and life long shoes.

As a new EMT, you quickly learn to manage complex calls and your ability to lead others comes more naturally. Over the years, you became accustomed to walking into any disaster, any tragic mess, and taking immediate charge. Rapidly determining what you have in front of you and taking action without an extra thought or moment's hesitation. You just make the event yours and others around you know that you took control for that specific reason. It was normally after the events or the call that you sat back and then it hit you what you just went through with your partner—that you just survived another one with only a few emotional scars. During the call, you are mentally taxed to your limit and often physically challenged but somehow you complete the call. More often than not, you were already exhausted and sleep deprived when the call came in. But you make it through the event and that's it. Any extra adrenalin is just enough to get your through until the event is over.

Although I was often emotionally scarred for some time after bad calls, it wasn't something you talked about with very many people. You had a few people you could trust to bare your soul to but that was rare. You never wanted to show anyone that you were weak or were just as scared as they were during the call. Some first responders are scarred for life because of the events they have to deal with. The dead kids and the mangled, burned bodies take their toll on everyone, no matter how long you have worked in EMS, heath care, or medicine.

In my experience, every staff member dealt with calls differently—some never showed that they were affected on the outside but they slowly changed. Some just up and quit one day, while others drank their pain away and increased their alcohol or drug use until they lost everything or committed suicide. Some people would think they were weak for quitting or walking away from it all, but if they only knew the pain and suffering they endured they, too, would have been overcome. After the very bad shifts or the bad calls I would sometimes cry, but not at the right times. Certain songs or circumstances would bring me back to the call or the events. Certain smells or sounds were not your friend.

To assume the role of an EMT, you need guts, determination and the stamina to do what others would not or could not do. Somedays you have to keep going no matter what gets thrown at you. I think Winston Churchill said it well when he proposed that "When you're going through hell, keep going." Grab on to your friends and your partners and take them with you. No one gets left behind. Even if they think they should just quit and die, bring them back from hell.

As an EMT, you need to face the fire and then walk right through it. Remember, you just need to get out before the devil knows that you were there. As time goes by, you learn to trust your instincts and go the extra mile for the right reasons. The right reasons are always the patients. EMS has a way of looking after you even if you aren't aware of it. There is always someone in your corner or on your side. You always have a "Rocky," pushing you ahead. The pictures I share are from a remarkable lady who knows pain and suffering I can't even imagine.

But not all days in EMS are bad or hard so don't think we work hard all the time. We had many days of nothing but too much coffee, extra sleep, no calls, and boredom beyond belief—and in seconds all hell would break loose and you'd get back at it. The time to yourself was time to contemplate the last call or the calls before, and this is how you achieved little chunks of wisdom along the way. Some days we would laugh and joke about the most trivial things we came across, all the while the people we were helping mattered, even if they were less fortunate than others. We would help them in times of need even if the calls were a result of being silly or doing things you would never admit to others. We made your day better and when we laughed, we laughed with you, never at you.

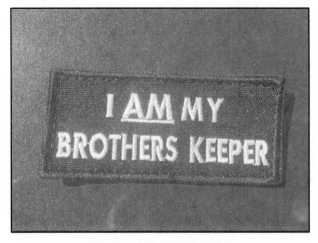

*My Reason is Simple: "You"*

Our days would sometimes seem very short and other times they would never end. You would learn to live with a full bladder, to be so dry you had trouble speaking, or so hungry, and then some days you would want to vomit at the sight of some very disgusting events or objects. You would constantly be learning, changing into a new uniform but not always having time to shower. Sometimes you forgot your watch at home, or you would be halfway to an emergency call and realize your glasses were at home still. You would learn to live with some people you loved and others you didn't like very much. You would have coworkers who didn't want to work EMS with you as they were there for the wrong reasons. But you made it through every call to the finish, in spite of all of it. You become a leader even if you were not born a leader or ever wanted to be one. You faced each day with a smile and you greeted the day with hope.

Your opinion mattered as you evolved and the more you learned in EMS, the more you become a real professional. Your long hard days were the ones that taught you the best lessons in life. Many of the lessons were hard on us but so much harder on the patients we were trying to help. Many died along the way despite our heroic efforts, but the lessons they taught us were simple in some ways and also very complex. But any lesson learned, even the little ones, are worthy of recounting.

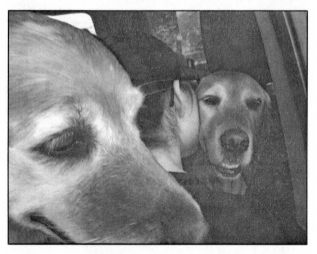

*"The people who mattered made it better in the end."*

*Chapter 3: Oxbow & Area Road Ambulance*

# "Character Building"

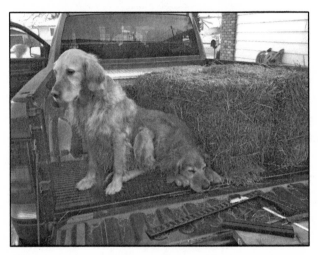

*"Building a Better Me"*

During my first introduction to EMS, I had the good fortune of starting in a rural service that was already ahead of the rest of the province in many ways. We had a good ambulance that had no real horsepower or no real ability to speed but was faithful. Even in the worst weather that Mother Nature could throw at us, we made it to the call and back again. As far as I can recall we never got stuck or stranded because of the weather. It would get so cold the light bar would stop rotating but that was optional anyway.

We had many close calls with wildlife, which was almost always white-tailed deer on the road or highway. I never hit one but a few times we were so close the hair likely stuck to the bumper. I'm sure someone was watching out for us as we had so many close calls but we were fortunate and never crashed or rolled a unit. We also had a few scary moments when we blew a tire while driving at high speed, which is scary enough.

Driving lights-and-siren was something I loved to do when it was required. But when you drive fast there is always less room for error and with error, death can be right next door. One tragic weekend I went to Oxbow and witnessed the effects of speed from the aftermath of a high-speed crash. A Trans Am that was driving around eighty miles an hour struck an RCMP cruiser on the driver's side. In the police car was Constable Butler whose RCMP cruiser was a complete mangled mess. The car was a mid-sized police cruiser with the widest part measuring not much more than three feet across. When I arrived, they were still taking him out and it was not easy or fast. The mess was horrific. Constable Butler died, whether from the initial crash or at the hospital, I can't remember. The driver of the Trans Am had his sternum go through the steering column. He was already dead on scene, as was his passenger. Alcohol and speed killed them all. It showed me speed wasn't always a good thing even as it related to EMS, and tonight it had killed everyone involved.

Actually, the closest I ever came to almost hitting and killing someone was in a high-speed chase years later that we came across in the middle of the night when I was working in Oxbow. It was during a blizzard in the middle of nowhere. So, you never knew what was coming and where the road would take you. You can plan many things but fate has its own agenda. You just need to always drive defensively and know that others on the road can and will kill you if you let them, so be prepared for anything. Never stop looking ahead and in all your fields of vision. You need to be ready for anything at any time as it isn't just your life at stake, but your partner's and the patient's, who are counting on you more than you could ever imagine.

We had many adventures and close calls but fate or destiny protected us from being in the path of harm's way. We ran out of gas for the longer transfers a few times and many times we had to plan our call to stop at an open gas station, which in the middle of Saskatchewan, in the middle of the night is not easy. Thankfully, we never had any great misadventures and we always made our trip with a story or two to tell the nurses after we got back from the calls. They never missed debriefing us or making us a warm coffee and showed us we mattered. They saved us more than once.

I started working in Oxbow when I was sixteen years old without even the right level of licence to drive for the first two years. I knew in my heart that EMS was where I was headed. I had no idea of what I was going to need to know to be successful but I was willing to do whatever it took to be the best to help our patients. I had the desire to stick it out even against the opposition and the trials from a society resistant to change. I had the basic desire to make a difference no matter what it took. I started working casually during the summer of 1982 and became full-time in March of 1983. Over the next years, we pushed the current staff and made our service even better than it was. When I left, it was state-of-the-art with very good equipment and very dependable educated staff working 24/7. By 1987 the Oxbow & Area Road Ambulance was one of the best EMS services in Saskatchewan and our staff proved it on every call. Allan or I were always just a call away and we never missed any bad calls or ignored the phone when someone needed help.

Most calls were what many would call routine. The calls were dispatched by the staff at Oxbow Union Hospital working on shift. I found out that many of these nurses who had been around for many years had more than experience to offer. They taught me compassion that only nurses know and will give out at no charge. Over the next several years we would see many tragedies and save a few lives together. The most important lesson I learned from the nurses was that everyone was unique and had different types of experience. We got to know our strengths and out weaknesses, which in turn made the team even more effective.

There were many days with no calls, but we had to keep the pager turned on at all times. The nurses were able to call us by phone when the pagers did not work. Looking back, we maybe only had about eight to twelve calls a month, but on many days the calls were challenging. We responded to emergency calls 24/7 and were expected to make the best out of every situation under all circumstances. Sometimes it meant using bystanders to drive, or farmers to help extricate a patient, or passing truckers to lift off vehicles when needed from the tragic events we came across. If we asked, people would help with no expectation of compensation. We got to see the best in people.

We provided a Basic Life Support (BLS) service at a high standard and strived to be the best of the best. We never said no to a call so if the phone rang we went, if someone needed help, we went, no matter how tired we thought we might be the next day. Nowadays, crews will time themselves out or choose not to respond for any possible reason they can find. It makes me so angry but I can't change the world. Just know when you're dedicated you find a way to respond. You make yourself available. You move the heavens and earth to help—even if the system doesn't care you still do and that is all that should matter.

We always had two people ready for calls and passed our pagers or radios around so the hospital or ambulance always had someone ready at a moment's notice. Allan, commonly known as "Bugs," or I tried to be on every call to ensure the care was the best it could be. On one of these days I was on a call with Barb, who was basically a driver with a Class 4 licence and had her first aid as well as the required CPR course. I was always the attendant on every call we did together and that was fine with me. Barb was a very dedicated and determined lady who would do what it took to make the call successful and we always got to our destination in one piece. This particular day, we got a call that a west-bound freight train had collided with a farm tractor at a level crossing. This is, to this day, one of the most horrific accidents involving a train and farm implements I have ever witnessed, and for that I'm grateful.

On the way to the scene we were told the patient was in cardiac arrest already so we came up with a great plan: Let's just grab him and get going to the local hospital as fast as humanly possible. The time on scene would be minimal. If there was any chance of getting him back, I thought, it was best that we get him to a doctor, pronto. Thinking about the facts and knowing the only real trauma hospital was at least two hours away was not encouraging. We had to get our game faces on as this was going to be a battle against death for sure. The odds were so against the patient living, and the reality of losing the battle was real and almost expected. We needed to get a patient breathing and a pulse back. Sounds easy if you're Superman, but Superman we were not. Still, we tried to fly anyway.

On arrival, we found a bystander and a local RCMP officer doing excellent CPR on the tractor driver. The tractor was in pieces, with parts of it on both sides of the train tracks and pieces of metal everywhere. The patient was lying close to the railroad tracks with two-man CPR in progress. I thought, "This is not going to be good" and was shocked when I reached over and found a pulse, and when they paused their chest compressions for the pulse check it was still present. Now my plan A was no good, as the patient was alive. Therefore, Plan B was now the best option, Airway, Breathing, Circulation (ABC), stabilization, and then get the heck off the scene but still in record time. It was just so unbelievable that anyone could survive or come back from that type of trauma. The tractor was so destroyed. It looked as if a missile had hit it. The patient should have been dead and why he now had a pulse was beyond my comprehension. Things just got a lot busier than we thought they would today. We became the team our patient needed and we made it work for our patient.

We elected to quickly package and get off the scene in record time, as we couldn't do much on scene that would help anyways. We just looked after the patient's airway and his pulse looked after itself. We had to perform frequent suctioning of the airway of copious amounts of blood to keep it clear, but still blood splattered everywhere. As well as trying to maintain an airway with a completely mangled patient with major airway complications, we also had multiple fractures to take care of, but we never really had enough hands to apply splints as we never got past the airway and breathing complications long enough. We headed to the closest hospital with a cool police escort that I completely missed. Later on, one of my friends told me that he watched us both go down Main Street and that it was the coolest thing he had ever seen. It was a pure mercy mission and we were doing our best regardless of the terror we faced. It was our battle to fight; it was the airway from hell and I wasn't going to lose.

Thank God, we patched the hospital en route and they were ready for us with the doctor and everyone at the ambulance bay, waiting. Once we got the patient inside the ER room, the hospital staff took over and they worked on trying to stabilize him. I went out and cleaned the back of the unit as best as possible. There was blood everywhere. In short time, the doctor came out and said to me, "Take him and go." He wanted us to load him up and make a mad dash for the next hospital that could do more for the patient than Oxbow could. We immediately took over again, grabbed an RN and took off.

We were travelling as fast as we could go with Barb fighting the traffic and ensuring we were safe. We worked so hard to keep the patient alive all while Barb drove as fast as possible. Unknown, mostly to me, we had a police escort again, which would have been cool to see if we weren't so busy in the back to notice. We were flying with amazing speed and cars were scattering out of our way to make our trip as fast as possible.

Before we had a chance to think about the huge mess we were involved in, we were rolling into St Joseph's Hospital in Estevan. We quickly unloaded and hospital staff took over and we had a chance to have a little break. We had made the second leg of our terrible trip without getting killed or harming anyone else. To our amazement and my utter shock, our patient was still fighting to live. I had no idea how a human body could take such punishment and still be able to maintain a pulse and have a BP we could measure. I had never seen so much blood leaking out of anyone who was still alive.

When we arrived in Estevan he was still fighting hard to live and the fact that he still had a pulse must have meant that we had been doing something right. Inside our unit, there was blood over everything, but worse than the last time. It was a huge mess of blood and body fluids. I started cleaning up the patient compartment one more time. We made the best of what we had in a short time to get it cleaned and ready to go again. This was while they were performing some very good emergency medicine on him to stabilize him to keep him alive for another trip—this one another ninety miles. It was not going to be a boring or uneventful transfer by any means.

We needed to take him on the next part of his journey right away so we had to get our crap together and be ready to work hard again. In a short time, his life would be ours again and we were already in way over our heads. We were only a BLS unit and any Advanced Life Support units (ALS) were not even close to us, so we had no other options. The patient was stabilized one more time by some of the best rural doctors and nurses in the world and we loaded up our patient and were off again.

The next stop was the Regina Plains Health Centre—our final destination—which was about another one-and-a-half hours away. It was the best hospital for this type of trauma but was so far away it seemed like a dream you could never reach. Barb was speeding along passing cars, passing semi-trucks and making the trip as straight as possible as she drove. If she were a poor driver, we would have been thrown around like sardines in a paint shaker.

We worked our magic and never quit until we got him inside the major trauma hospital and he was still alive. We transferred care for the last time and I was completely exhausted. Barb must have been just as spent as I was as she had been a miracle driver, fighting traffic for hours and making our trip as safe as possible. That was what teams do: we worked together and we got the work done no matter what. I went out to the unit and almost cried. There was blood on the ceiling, the walls and the floor were moving with blood and IV fluid. I'd never seen such a mess in my life. This was the third time I'd have to clean the unit on the same call and I was done.

I went and asked the janitor for a mop and a pail. He looked at me and said, "Son, you go have a coffee. I got this one." I was in disbelief as I had no idea he could or would help us. We went and sat down for a bit and just started talking about our past six or seven hours of hell. Sometimes the people who save us are those who are put on this earth for a special reason, and in this case that person was a janitor who earned the least amount of money of anyone working in that entire hospital. Barb and I got a coffee and had time to recharge enough to realize we had survived hell.

We were still covered in blood ourselves as we had no clean clothes and it didn't faze us in the least as we returned to our unit. When we opened the back door to assess the damage, I was speechless. To this day, I still have trouble believing it. Our patient compartment was cleaned to a new level and there was no evidence of the mess we just had endured for the last terrible hours. That janitor was our angel. He had performed a miracle that day.

We were out of service as we were missing so many supplies, but the mess was gone. To this day, that man is my personal hero. Looking back, he was just part of the team. That day, he saved a life just as effectively as the rest of us.

Barb and I then realized we had both left in a hurry so many hours ago with no money, and we hadn't had a chance to eat for many hours. Thankfully, one of the nurses made our day by giving us some money for food that saved us one more time that day. Then we started our way back home and started to debrief ourselves on what we had just gone through. We made it home with food and coffee in us, which was well past due. That call took a lot out of us, but it also affected everyone involved in the patient's care despite the outcome in the days to come. From the accident scene to everyone involved in his hospital care, people did their best.

Looking back, I sometimes can't understand how we made it through that day and, especially, how our patient could live as long as he did with such severe and ultimately fatal injuries. He lived for another five days and then his battle was over. He was just too broken to go on. We did our best to stabilize him but the secondary injuries and cellular insult that occurred after the initial injury must have been horrific.

Tragically, his family's struggle with the outcome would last much longer. I went to his memorial service with my mum and met some of his family members. They were so appreciative and all came over to thank me for doing our best. Unbeknownst to me at the time we had received our family Border collie from his parents. Several of our previous dogs were also from his family over the years. They were well-known breeders of some of the best herding dogs in the province. Their family had known my parents before I was even born. I had even watched his brother on TV as a kid, never realizing one day I would try so hard to save his close family member.

This was just one of the many times when we would be called to a fatal or near-fatal event. So many times, you would see tragic accidents with only minor injuries but the next time the vehicles would be a mangled mess and the victim would be dead. There was no way to predict the outcomes as there were so many factors that you had no control over. The things we learned to be the best predictors of a bad outcome were simple and almost always present in the dispatch information. This was followed by the mechanism of injury (MOI), which always followed the law of physics, which in most cases we could not alter but we still somehow managed to defeat from time to time. Thinking back, some people just wouldn't die and others wouldn't live despite any rules or laws.

Motorbike accidents (MBA) were almost always bad, whereas with a single vehicle rollover (SVR), you would never know until you arrived on scene. The one event that always had a bad outcome was the farming accidents. Those never had people with minor injuries. From a crushed pelvis to missing arms and legs, it was not uncommon to see death and tragedy affect people that you knew or cared about in some way. Over time, you got to know many of the people in your community and in the surrounding communities.

We also did our fair share of transfers and responded to calls for elderly patients who had fallen and broken a leg, or sadly, their hip or pelvis at the same time. It was common to find some patients a day or two after the fall. Sadly, we had little to offer them for pain until Entonox become available, and it couldn't be used six to eight months of the year as it separated very quickly in the cold Canadian climate.

We also picked up many sick elderly patients only to find out a few hours later they had expired. It was an eerie feeling knowing a few hours ago, you were talking to them and they were having their last ride on earth and soon they would be gone from this world. They would be taking so many memories with them that would never be shared again. Many of these patients had increased shortness of breath (SOB), silent heart attacks and, looking back, they most likely had what we called a type 2 acute myocardial infarction (AMI). Essentially this means that their heart was pushed so hard it just couldn't take the extra workload and eventually failed physically or structurally.

On reflection, over the years I think that working in my home town pushed me even harder than others I'm sure. Working with the Oxbow & Area Road Ambulance also pushed me to be even better than I could ever imagine. Thanks to Allan Needham, Len Yates, Tanis MacRae for always believing in me and pushing me to take the next steps in my education. I started with so little knowledge; I lacked the essential common sense and had no idea of the big picture of the real emergency medicine world. My learning was never-ending and every day I became a better person regardless of where I had come from. It didn't matter; after I got going I would not be stopped. The more you learn the more you realize you don't know enough and the cycle just continues as you evolve into your final attainment in your career I found out over time.

I was so fortunate to work with such good people and, over time, we made the service an incredible service and the patients and community became our pride. They wanted us if they ever needed an ambulance and they went the extra mile for us. Just as we went the extra mile for them when they needed us the most. We formed lifelong friendships despite the hardships we faced.

My biggest regret in my life is not being able to go back and work as a paramedic in Saskatchewan, but some things just aren't meant to happen. The community only knew a Basic Life Support (BLS) service, and an Advanced Life Support (ALS) service wasn't going to make it to the small towns for all the wrong reasons. Everyone wanted a doctor even if they were not very good, but they didn't want or wouldn't pay for an ALS service even if we could save lives or make it more of an efficient health care system.

It would simply cost too much to have a paramedic, which I and many others know is so backwards, but the way many people felt at the time just the same. It would not be for many years that Shock Trauma Air Rescue Society (STARS) finally arrived in Saskatchewan. One day my mum called me, excited, and told me that STARS had landed within a few miles of our family farm and helped save a life. The fact that an ALS service had made it to our remote area meant that it now could and would be able to happen.

Knowing that ALS can at least fly to where I started my career is so amazing, but also surreal to me. I can now sleep much better knowing that my immediate family and friends have that service available to them. Thank you, STARS. It is now some twenty years since I was a STARS nurse in Alberta, and back then I didn't believe I would see this happen in my lifetime. My mum was able to see the STARS helicopter use our farm as a landmark, just as the planes and jets had for years when we were kids watching them fly over our heads.

STARS would now be able to help people like Jamie, and even Burt, who could have been given an honest chance if ALS was available. If we had ALS back then, and I was there knowing what I know today, I would have kicked the angel of death's ass right out of the ambulance and Burt would have lived.

Thinking back, one of the best things about Oxbow was the nurses I worked with. I spent many hours at the hospital in the middle of the night, helping them to lift or turn patients and keep the nurses safe when trouble was around. There was one time, in particular, that I felt extremely grateful that they had my number. I was home sleeping and was awakened by the phone ringing. The nurses were calling for help right away. I threw on some clothes and was out the door in a minute. My window was frozen over with ice and snow on it so seeing wasn't going to be easy. I put my side window down and took off for the hospital as fast as I could drive. On arrival, the RCMP cruiser was parked by the front door and the nurses were standing outside waving frantically. "He's killing him!" they said. I hit the hospital doors running, and as soon as I got into the front lobby I found the fight. Ralph, one of the local RCMP officers, was fighting for his life with a monster of a man. He must have been about six-foot-six and a very big man. I think Ralph was trying to get his gun out to shoot him but couldn't get his hand free. I just lunged for his assailant's head and neck and got a hold of him and took him down and it was over in seconds. I knew that in a fight if you got ahold of the head and neck of any person or animal, you always won. I just couldn't break someone's neck or smash their head into the wall or floor on the way down, or I'd be in much more trouble than I was looking for. As soon as he was pinned down, Ralph got the guy handcuffed and we escorted him out to the police car. Ralph must have called a 10-33, which means officer in trouble, as police cars were coming from the closest detachments almost sixty miles away.

Ralph asked me if I could help take the guy to the local jail and get him booked in. I said sure. The nurses would find someone to cover me if there was an ambulance call. So, we were off. The funny thing was once we got him into the cell, the guy started crying. I'd never seen such a big man cry so much. Honestly, he kept saying, "I want my mommy." Well, sorry to tell you, big guy, but your situation was way beyond anything Mommy could fix. He was going to do some jail time and, more important, sober up. Then just maybe he would stop acting like a baby, even if he was past the diaper stage by some twenty odd years.

This was just a normal day in Oxbow; you just never knew what was going to happen next. I was somedays a mechanic, a welder, a mortician's assistant to police officer's backup in a dire emergency.

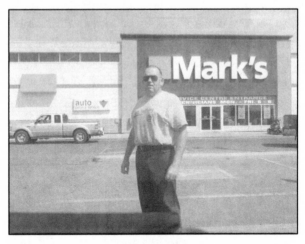

*"Tough Enough"*

*"I would always stand up for the people who needed it the most. I would not be bullied after my high school days. We did what we could and God only knows how many times we almost got hurt."*

## Chapter 4: The Race to Save Burt
# "The Day the Music Died"

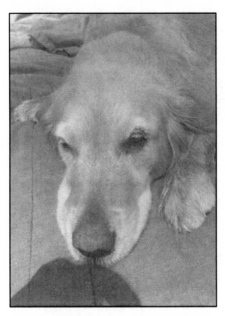

*"Saving Just One at All Costs"*

There are days that you never want to repeat, and this was one day that I will never forget. Saskatchewan has days when driving conditions and visibility can be good one minute and terrible the next. This particular day, the roads were treacherous at best. We prairie folk were accustomed to adverse weather, but even then, bad things would still happen. It always seemed to me as though bad accidents tended to happen to good people. Some amazing people I've known over the years have been killed this way.

I lost my uncle, Bill Bayliss, and my cousin Darryl in one day from exposure to hydrogen sulfide gas. It broke my grandma's heart. I also lost a childhood friend, Rodney Carnduff, who was killed in a single-car rollover. Looking back, it was a preventable death. Rodney had spent the summer running the New Holland Bale Wagon, our 1049 hay bale stacker. I was too young to drive it but I knew what levers to pull and we made a good team. He could reach the operational pedals and I could fit to his side like a glove. We made hauling bales so easy.

The race to save Burt will likely always stand out as one of the worst days of my life. These are the days that will either make or break us in spite of the help or the support we get from our friends and EMS family. I will never forget that day, but I also know I can't change the past no matter how much I'd like to. Even still, I fight that battle over and over again in my mind, though the outcome is always the same. From the very start of this very tragic call I never knew it was Burt until it was too late or the call was over. Looking back what happened that day was something that will haunt me for life even if it was not my fault. I will bear the pain.

I was working as a mechanic and a welder at the time to support my mere existence, as EMS pay wasn't very good, but it was the best we could hope for in the early days. We lived by the radio and the phones as a secondary backup on every shift. The nurses always knew how to find us, or at least one of us. Our radios came to life that terrible day with the nurses calling for the ambulance to attend to a single vehicle rollover west of Highway 9, just past the junction on Highway 18. The cause of the accident was as expected being the terrible roads and black ice that was so common in this type of weather. It was already a terrible day to drive, with the current road conditions getting worse by the hour. We scrambled to get to the base and were off as fast as we could safely travel. We had to make it to the scene safely, as we were the only help the injured would have for miles. I would go from fixing a farm implement to saving a life in minutes those days, and the latter were much more complex in most cases.

When the call came in, I had no idea it would change me forever. The outcome was so tragic for so many people that day. I could not pray after the fact that Burt had had better winter tires or that his speed might have been less, but I did anyway. The truth was Burt was doomed from the start, as soon as his vehicle lost control.

If only we had been an Advanced Life Support (ALS) unit that day, maybe we could have helped. But our level of care was only Basic Life Support (BLS). More important, the circumstances were the perfect receipt for a complete disaster. Everything was set up perfectly for someone to lose their life this day.

Upon arrival, we found a vehicle that had been rolled in the north ditch. Bystanders were trying to help someone in the bottom of the snow-covered ditch. Initially, I thought we only had one patient and it would be okay, as another apparent victim was walking around and looked uninjured. That person was my friend Tom. I'd known Tom for years as he was my eldest brother's best friend. I then noticed one of the local hospital staff trying to help a patient lying in the snow. The patient I didn't recognize was Burt, who appeared to be having a grand mal seizure and had his teeth clenched and no effective airway. I quickly went to his side and tried to help using simple ABC methods. All we knew was we needed an airway; we also needed an effective breathing depth and an adequate heart rate. Finally, we needed a palpable pulse. No matter what order they were in, or if you worked on them simultaneously, all these things had to be addressed and fixed if they weren't adequate.

No matter how hard I tried that day I could not get an oral pharyngeal airway (OPA) to establish a patent airway. Sadly, we had no nasal pharyngeal airway (NPA) and I could tell Burt's air exchange was next to none. I couldn't get past the airway problem. I almost got my finger taken off trying to open his mouth enough to get in any size of an airway. It wouldn't help, as he was clenched so tight. We applied high flow oxygen, a cervical collar, and then log rolled him onto a long spine board and took him directly to the unit. The hospital was about seven to ten minutes away. I knew they would help and they had many more options that I did in our BLS unit. We just had to make a mad dash for some ALS care. We wasted no time at all on scene. But time was so against us we never had a chance. Destiny was making its case for us to lose no matter what, as everything was going wrong that day.

When we reached the unit, Burt was done having his seizure. We then lost his pulse and the clock had run out on his poor life even with our best intentions. All we could do was perform CPR and that seemed so helpless. It should not have come to this, but it did.

I suspected his death was likely related to the blow to the head he'd endured and the hypoxia that came immediately after. It was most likely related to poor perfusion as well as a hypoxic brain inducing the seizure, which I had thought right away was caused by a significant head injury. On one of the rolls, Burt was likely partially out the side window with his chest and head exposed, and he was struck between the snow-covered ground and the truck. The MOI was severe. There were no obvious major external injuries. I just couldn't get past the airway on my assessment treatments. We always use an ABC approach and fix what we find along the way. But when you have a bad airway, it's not a good idea to go directly to breathing as it's not going to get any better without a patient airway. Then without effective breathing, everything gets worse by the second.

We patched the hospital to let them know we were about seven minutes away with an adult male now in cardiac arrest. I kept thinking over and over that we needed a damn airway right from the start. A hypoxic seizure is almost impossible to interrupt unless you can break the cycle. This might have been possible with ALS medications but we had none and no one to administer them. So, looking back, Burt was doomed right from the start and no matter what we did or couldn't do, his fate was already determined. After you go into traumatic cardiac arrest, you almost never have a chance of survival even if you're in a trauma room with the best of the best fighting for your life.

When it comes to the golden hour, we could not have done anything different during our time on scene, which is commonly referred to as the platinum ten minutes. Once we were in transport and Burt was in cardiac arrest, we could open his airway and ventilate, but it was too late to save the brain cells. His heart was already compromised and had stopped. His brain was already past any form of auto-regulation. It was shut off. I was scrambling and looking at him and wondering what else can we do?

I still had not recognized at the time that the patient we were so desperately trying to save was Burt. We worked hard to maintain an airway, used the OPA, used our suction and did CPR as best as we could, as it was all we could do. We had no ALS care, we had no cardiac monitors. We had no specialized equipment to assess the patient's oxygen levels known as a $SpO_2$ monitor or a carbon dioxide ($CO_2$) monitor. We had no Automatic External Defibrillator, and it wouldn't have been helpful in a trauma arrest anyway. All we had going for us was that it was going to be a witnessed arrest.

There were no drugs involved in the accident, and no one could blame alcohol. The accident was purely due to the terrible weather conditions.

Upon arrival at Oxbow hospital, we unloaded as fast as we could and one staff member walked Tom into the hospital while the rest of us kept doing CPR and headed for the old under-equipped ER room. We gave a quick verbal report to the nurse and the doctor on the way. The on-call doctor walked in and quickly assessed Burt and called the time of death. I could not believe it. We only did CPR for ten minutes in total. We never started an IV, we never gave any epinephrine, intubated or attempted to capture an airway. I thought he had a chance in my heart. How could we not do anything? I was shocked and didn't know what to say. I felt lost.

We just lost another one and nothing would change it now. I thought maybe we could have done something more. There had to be something more we could have done. Why did Burt need to die? He had so many years of life left in him.

I then composed myself and walked out of the trauma room and found his friend Tom in the X-ray room. Tom looked at me as I walked up. He knew the outcome already; you could see it in his eyes. I said, "Tom your friend is dead—he didn't make it." He looked at me and said, "That's not my friend. That's Burt." I couldn't tell you the shock and horror I felt at that moment. I had no idea it was Burt until that second. How the hell did I miss that? I'd known Burt for years. Tom was my brother's best friend and I'd known him for years. Burt was a great person and an all-around nice person. Tom would not hurt anyone. Now he was dead from a freak accident on a patch of bad road.

Just a few weeks before the accident we were sitting having a beer together and Burt looked at me and said he could never do my job. I told him I loved it and it was so much better than anything I'd ever done before. I told him I loved the farm but this was where I could help the most. Burt was a farmer and a musician. I said to him that my life had a purpose now and I needed that. Now this... What could I say? I hadn't recognized him until it was too late. I should have known it was Burt. He wasn't very broken or that bloody, but I always knew him with thick glasses and he just didn't look the same without them. Maybe my brain blocked it on purpose. Burt was an amazing human being. He was a gifted musician. A truly gifted guitar player gone just like that and we couldn't save him. Just like that he was dead.

If only I had recognized him, I just might have done an emergency cricothyrotomy and lost my licence gladly or taken my chances if only he could live. Why didn't I recognize him, I thought over and over? Why didn't the on-call doctor do more, I thought? But I already know the answer to that unspoken question. He was not trained. He was a small-town rural doctor and was not trained in trauma care. He lacked the proper emergency training that was mandatory in many urban centres and it was not his fault at all. Emergency medicine was a relatively new specialty back then. Nothing was to change the outcome of that day, but I had no idea the worst was yet to come.

Over the next days and weeks, my life would become hell. The family was told that if I had just done my job, Burt would have lived. They told him I should have done a surgical airway procedure. That would be correct if I was a paramedic or a trauma doctor, but I was not trained for the skill at all. Why they blamed me I will never know but, in hindsight, they needed someone to blame so if it was to be me then so be it. I would take the blame even if it was wrong.

I'm sure from that day forward after the accident, there were bad feelings toward me from Burt's family, despite our families being close. Even though I hadn't made the road conditions so terrible, or made them lose control, or made him roll and then be ejected without seat belts. I would never have coffee in their home again. I would never be able to joke with Burt's dad or brother again. When I looked at his mother, I would just see a great sadness that I could never help.

Over the years, I took on the souls of many who were lost. I came to realize that was okay as that was who I was on the inside and what made me unique. Later in life, my friend and pastor, John Anderson, gave me some good advice. "God only deals us as much pain as we can carry," he said. If people truly knew me, they would know I wasn't someone to just do enough. I always gave my patients

110 percent. I could never do a half-assed job. I would not have let Burt die if I could have prevented it.

I lost that battle with Burt in more ways than you can imagine. Thankfully, I could just add it to my list of misfortune and keep crawling ahead. Somedays it felt as if I was drowning and had no one to turn to, but I had no choice but to not look back. So, trudge on ahead, I did, even if I didn't know which direction I was heading. As long as you have some fight left in you, you must be alive, I thought. This one event knocked me down and, somehow, I had to get back up. I got up and finished the fight, even knowing I'd already lost it.

After that day, I was different and never will be the same person again but I was not beaten. I knew there had to be a better way. Sometimes you have to be knocked to the ground and feel pain in order to get back up at all. Life can work that way somedays. Life is so precious and we can only do our best and what happens will happen.

Once a bad event occurs, the initial injury is often the main thing we can't change or fix. I took some time and thought about what I could and could not change. I could not go back and change the outcome of the accident but I could change my future by changing me. I wanted to be a paramedic. I could never be a doctor even if I wanted to, as I was a grade ten dropout.

I thought that nursing would be a great entry into the medical profession. Paramedics were not common in rural locations. Only urban centres could train or use them, which limited where I could live. Plus, you had to have more education than I had at the time to be a paramedic, so nursing seemed like the best fit.

It was my friends that saved me from the terrible nightmares and terrible thoughts I had following Burt's death. Good people will die and bad people will live; it's not our call or decision to make as to who lives and who doesn't. It's in God's hands.

I would show everyone who ever tried to knock me down that I had what it took. I came across a good tattoo on a very wise lady that plainly read, "If you get knocked down seven times, get up eight times." Well, I knew a thing or two about being knocked down. I just needed to get the hell up and put my head and mind on a better path in life. That was for me to do, no one else. I had one or two more fights left in me so they had better not try to bury me just yet. I wasn't done the battle; it was just the end of the round.

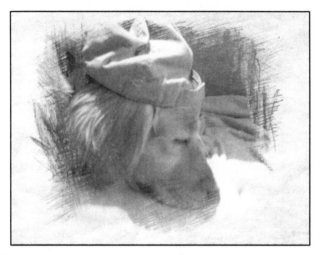

*"Somedays the people around you are the only ones who matter."*

*Chapter 5: Stepping Up to the Plate*

# "Making It Better
# Than It Was"

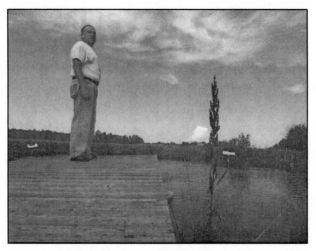

*"Making a Change in Just One Day"*

The time to step up to the plate was now, as far as I was concerned. I had no idea the depth of knowledge that RNs had was so diverse, and the learning curve was as steep as life itself. The more I learned, the more I realized I didn't know anything at all.

I had to say goodbye to Burt and move on with my life. I knew in my heart that his death wasn't my fault even if some people were blaming me. If I had of gone beyond my scope of practice, I'd never work in EMS again.

I signed up to write the GED to get a grade twelve equivalency, and I was trying to get out of my poor frame of mind. That night a good friend and I had way too much to drink and went to the cemetery to say goodbye to Burt. The goodbyes were permanent. I said my piece and left it up to a higher power and Burt to accept my apologies.

The next day I had a small problem. I couldn't legally drive yet and I had five exams to write. I called a good friend and explained my predicament. Within a few minutes, I had a driver and we were off. I made it through the first three exams and my head never exploded but it sure felt close. For lunch, I had an emergency bottle of Coke and two aspirin and did two more exams without remembering much about any of them. I just knew I had the worst headache of my life, but it was my own fault. Not my finest moment. But somehow, I had to get over a very bad time in my life. Pain is good sometimes. With pain, you feel something and if you feel pain you're still alive, so all hope is not lost.

A few weeks later, I got my marks and they called me with the good news. I said no way could those be my results as I was not capable of such high marks. The woman on the phone verified my social insurance number and, sure enough, they were my marks. My principal in high school and few of the teachers had made it very clear I was a nothing. I had no idea how this was possible.

Maybe it was Burt or Jamie showing my pen what answer to circle, but I'm certain even to this day that I didn't earn those marks on my own. They were both very good students and gifted in almost everything. However, I managed it, I had crossed the first hurdle to get into nursing school, and I was ready for the next part of my life. My biggest lessons so far were that you have to let go of the bad in your life to move on. Then you have to make good out of what's left of the broken pieces. Even if you're beaten and broken, you're still alive. If you think you have nothing, but you feel pain, it's a start. With pain, at least you know you're alive, and it's all I had left in those days. Now, I had the marks to get into nursing school. I just had to figure out how to get there somehow.

I had a few months to get my stuff ready, and the first but also the biggest problem was getting out of my comfort zone. I had some serious soul-searching to do. Basically, I had to somehow convince myself I could do it. Too often, I had vivid flashbacks of my high school principal coming up to me and saying, "You're a Bayliss—you should quit today." He was a terribly poor role model as a person. The scary thing was that he was in a position of power and was supposed to be there to help build students up but he didn't care about us. He had no idea how hard I worked or how much I cared about other people.

I would show him what it took to be a leader of people. I had a flashback of my mum standing up for me one day in the principal's office and telling him exactly what she thought of him, using some very colourful language. I was so proud of my mum that day. Well, if my mum thought I could be somebody, to hell with him. I was thinking that if my dad was there, he would have knocked him out cold and wouldn't even have broken a sweat. Dad could move faster than Superman. He was ten of our principal in one.

I would show him that despite being written off because of my last name I was more then he would ever be in his whole entire life. I would show him that I had the guts, the wisdom and the dedication to be one of the best of the best. From that day forward, I would make sure that the people under my watch were treated right. They could always count on me and my word would be paid with blood if needed.

I had to resign from my position as the manager for the Oxbow & Area Road Ambulance and they hired someone to replace me and that was that. I had no regrets about leaving for a better education and to make a difference in my patients' lives, but the move and the loss of working with so many good people was hard for me. I will always be thankful to the people like Len and Cathy, who kept me out of trouble while I was working some days without much sleep.

Len had operated the local ambulance for years, as well as running the funeral home, and thankfully he was the manager at the Massey Ferguson dealership and made my days go by better than expected more often than not. So, leaving Oxbow also meant leaving a good part-time job where there was always something to fix or put together. Only once did I miss work as I was so tired that I'd passed out for at least sixteen hours after working two or three days with barely any sleep. I made it to work the next afternoon in time for afternoon coffee. Len stood up for me and told my boss I needed the rest. Len had seen me going hard for days and had listened to me during the night on the scanner. He knew every time I had a call and understood that my being available to help people when I was needed was what mattered the most.

Thankfully, I had my dad and my mum to help me get to Regina, and they made sure I never starved and had enough gas money to come home on the weekends. So, off I went to a new world and away from my comfort zone. To a big city and an adventure that I would never have dreamed of, coming from a farm and being a farm kid at heart for all my life.

The day I left Oxbow was sadder than most days but also rewarding, for in my mirror I could see the sunrise and ahead of me I could see the future—but better yet I could see the wide-open blue sky. Somedays you just have to drive away, and your brain can tell your broken heart it is the right thing to do.

# "Just a Nurse"

My enrollment to nursing school was just like everything else that I had done in my life. It was not straightforward and the first day was just as strange. Looking back, I knew I would be looking at a personal challenge and I wasn't let down. I had to ask myself why I wanted it so bad and the answer was simple as life itself. In order to save lives, I had to know more. As an EMT, I had basic life support knowledge as well as some very good basic skills, but people were dying in spite of my best intentions. I needed more training and this was my next step to a higher education.

I was reminded often that Burt had died partly from my lack of advanced skill, so mastering the skills needed to make it so others would live under such horrific circumstances was mandatory and not an item on a wish list.

I walked into the Saskatchewan Institute of Applied Arts and Technology SIAST and was amazed at the number of students in the building. Some, like me, were also associate studies students, who lacked the initial marks or entrance requirements. There were about 300 to 400 students in the building at the Parkway Campus. I met with a counsellor and was shocked to find out that someone was giving me a chance that I never thought possible. They had some extra spots in the psychiatric nursing program and they would consider me for one of the spots if I was interested. But I had no real savings and I had planned to work part-time to put myself through school. I called my dad and he said to do it. So, my first day I went from being a part-time student to a full-time student. SIAST had given me my chance to get ahead despite my terrible past academic history.

I worked hard for the first semester and my practical days were easier than I thought because I had worked EMS. I had mastered the first part of nursing, which was essentially how to talk to patients and how to make their day better. I kept checking my marks and was shocked time and again. Even though a number of my classmates quit or failed, I stayed in the race. All I had to do was to keep going. Everything was going so well and then I ran into another huge roadblock.

I was living with my brother and he decided he wasn't ready for school, packed up and went home. I had no extra money and could not afford the apartment by myself. So, I needed to come up with a backup plan or I was doomed. I talked to my friend Tanis and she said, "You're moving in with my parents," and that was that. I had no idea who they were or what they did, and boy was I in for shock. They turned out to be brilliant people, both highly educated, dedicated and very family-oriented. They welcomed me into their home, and every day I spent there was a blessing. I never felt unwanted or in the way and I always knew I could tell them anything and they would listen, and together we would come up with a plan. I made them proud. That mattered to me more than life itself some days.

I could not believe how fast nursing school was going by and was amazed by some of my instructors as they were true mentors. One of the best I remember was Pam: she was so kind and caring and had a way of making you feel better about yourself. When you had a good instructor, your patients were better off, your education was more rewarding and you excelled in clinical rotation. Other instructors were not as kind and a few didn't think males should be in nursing. We started with around thirty male students and only nine of us graduated; I was one of the fortunate ones still around at graduation.

We had shared a lot of laughs in nursing school, and there were a few times when my patients rendered me speechless. This one patient was trying his best to stand and void at the urinal. I was at his side to keep him standing long enough to get the job done. He looked down, then he looked at me, then he looked down again and shook his head. Then he said to me, "Eighty years of shit and abuse and it just shriveled up to nothing." I didn't say anything. What can you say to that? Sometimes a response is not required.

You can't take life too seriously all the time. After all, no one gets out alive anyway. We need to make the most of every second we're here and look for the humour in every situation. Even when our day is not going our way, we can find something good in the world. We often measure a person solely based on his bad behaviour, when he may have made many positive contributions to society. People need to be forgiven for their mistakes and let God be the judge.

By the end of our second year I faced another hurdle in school. I had one low mark and it was a hard class. Without the right grade, I wasn't going to continue as a full-time student. I was working too much, I know, and I had that going against me. Many people at school didn't know that at the time I was working all night a seniors' group home and then going to class during the day. I was lucky to get a few hours' sleep before and after classes, and off I'd go. It helped pay my tuition, but when it came to concentrating and doing my school work, it was difficult.

In addition to going to school and working, I had some weekends off so I would go home and help my dad on the farm. This also cut into my study and homework time greatly. The night before the exam, I crammed like crazy and went through a few cans of Jolt cola. There was a Timmy's nearby, and that helped me to stay alert and awake, as well. The next day I went and did the exam. I had to wait a while for my marks, and when they came back and were higher than I expected, I was so happy. From that day forward, I worked less on the side and did more homework and made school my main focus. My dad helped me financially, as well, and I got a student loan which made life much easier. I had to pick my battles and this was one battle I had to win. My new profession was not something I was taking lightly.

My second year went by in a flash, and before I knew it we were getting ready to graduate. The past two years were a blur of good times and hard times, but it was so fulfilling to know that I was achieving a goal and my life would soon get a lot better. Once I graduated, I was going to face my next hurdle in life and the sky was still blue. I just had to make the best choices and make my education count. I had made some very good friendships in nursing school but sadly after we graduated, we all went our separate ways in life and today I only know of a few of my classmates. We started with about 240 students and about 130 graduated, which was a significant loss. In the beginning, all I wanted was to finish so I could walk away knowing I had made it this far and my life was just starting all over again. As it turned out, I excelled in many things and I had exceeded in the goals I set out to achieve. I had made the grades, passed my clinical rotations, met my graduation requirements and, in June 1989, I walked across the stage as a grade ten dropout with a GED to becoming a registered nurse.

I also had a job waiting for me. I had nowhere to live but decided I would just find a place when I got to Wetaskiwin, Alberta. I had applied for the job at a career event in Saskatoon and received a call before I got back to Regina that I had a job offer.

I had applied for one other job but never got an interview and, sadly, it was because I was a male nurse. It kind of shocked me, but I had faced discrimination several times as a nurse already. When I was visiting with the SIAST school nurse, I told her about the situation and she made a few phone calls. Unbeknownst to me, she was very up on rules and regulations. I also found out she was on the Saskatchewan Union of Nurses as a committee member. I guess I talked to the right person that day. The person who made that decision to not hire me was terminated and they offered me the job the next day. But I was reluctant to pack up and move somewhere that I might not be wanted. If they didn't want me the first time, I wasn't going to take the chance of walking into an already unhealthy new job and setting myself up for failure.

Looking back, had I stayed in Saskatchewan I wouldn't have had the same opportunities for additional education and the ability to go as far as I did in the Alberta EMS system. At the time, the two provinces were so different than they are today. Over the last five or more years, they have become much closer in terms of the level of education and pay, as well as the increased complex ALS care now arriving in Saskatchewan EMS. When STARS went to Saskatchewan, the level of care improved all across the province. At that time, in 1989, I think the average nurse was paid about seven dollars more an hour in Alberta, which after some time adds up nicely.

It was so amazing. I went from being paid $1.56 an hour to making approximately thirty dollars an hour after just a few years' education. Life had thrown me some crazy curveballs but somehow, I had managed to anchor myself to my future.

My days in nursing school were over. I had to get out of my comfort zone again, and start over again in a new career. The starting over was very exciting and scary all at the same time. The hardest part was moving even farther away from my friends in Oxbow and my family.

My real learning was about to start and I had no idea how little I knew. I would slowly learn that medicine is so vast and the EMS world is so complex. The funny thing was that nursing was my field but not my chosen profession. Even today I'm not really happy with my College & Association of Registered Nurses of Alberta (CARNA), which was my provincial leaders or body of nursing that are accountable for our overall registration and practice of care, as they have let me down over and over again, but my nursing colleagues are some of the best people in the world. In the end, I can't blame anyone but myself.

I just had to avoid looking back at everything I was leaving behind. That was the hardest part of it all. I had the pain from my past pushing me ahead to the destiny I could only achieve if I took the plunge into the big unknown.

## Chapter 7: Alberta Bound
# "A Year Becomes a Lifetime"

Graduation was in the big picture and I needed a paying job. I had looked around Saskatchewan and there were no good opportunities that suited me. I filled out an application for Wetaskiwin General Hospital (WGH) in Alberta, as they were looking for registered nurses. I had no idea where Wetaskiwin was or anything about the type of hospital it was. I had no idea then that it would be where I would start my real training. I would see more complex situations there than most people could ever imagine.

I had no idea when I came to Alberta that I was never going to return to Saskatchewan to work. I was offered a job at WGH in Emergency, with some operating room (OR) on-call; it was a full-time position and I would be starting within a few weeks. I knew I had to make a go of it. I had applied to a few jobs in Saskatchewan and was not sure where that would take me so I said yes. July 4, 1989, proved to be my first day as a paid nurse. I had my dad's support and my brother Donnie helped move my stuff to Wetaskiwin and also helped move two other nurses' belongings in the trailer as we all graduated together and had jobs within one hundred miles of each other in Alberta. I had a special song picked out for our drive, and as we rumbled out of Regina, Saskatchewan, I turned it on and turned it up. The song was simple but said a lot to me. It was "Someday" by Steve Earl. It simply said there isn't a lot you can do in this small town, which to me was Oxbow, Saskatchewan.

If I wanted to get somewhere I had to go down that road to a better place and that had to be a long way away. Not my choice, maybe, but a job was a job. I thought about the song and it said what I was feeling all too well: "Someday I'm going to get out of here." It meant so much to me, personally. I'd never had much luck, so I had to make my own. The saddest thing for me was leaving behind Tanis and the MacRae family who had taken me in and raised me for the last one-and-half years. They had given me hope and a desire to be more than I ever could be where I was in my current career and with my life. Now, I would truly be on my own, on the right path for my future life.

Over the next day, we all got moved to Alberta. Wetaskiwin had a population of about 10 000, and I was amazed at how big it was. Oxbow had about 1200 people with some smaller towns and villages that made up our service area. I found a very nice apartment and got moved in and then I had to find everything I needed to function. Everything from the hospital to the local stores, and I needed to get a bank account so I could be paid, which Maureen from the credit union arranged. She was the most wonderful lady and for the next fifteen years she was always only a phone call away. Maureen helped me with everything from loans to emergency money, to finding anything I needed that I was lost finding. She was truly a lifesaver in my life for many years.

Wetaskiwin (and Wetaskiwin General) was a very busy place, with an increased amount of crime, accidents, overdoses, severe beatings and just about anything you could imagine at any given time when you got to work. We bordered on five neighbouring First Nations reserves and had to pick up patients there at times, as well when there were no other ambulances available. I was completely shell-shocked to learn about three unrelated murders in and around my new home city in the first couple of weeks after I moved there. The orientation to the hospital was great and the staff was amazing. Joyce Nelson was the head of the education department and she run a very good effective department. We also staffed three ambulances as well as we were expected to work our shifts as Emergency Room (ER) nurses. One of the ER nurses was always the attendant on any ambulance call, with one Licensed Practical Nurse (LPN) or a Nursing Attendant as the driver for every call. So, in addition to staffing up to 3 EMS units we also were staffing the crazy emergency room that never slept. We got to learn to run, drink coffee and start IV's in a hurry.

It was essentially a scoop-and-run service for the most part as we had to get our patients back to the ER where we always had other patients waiting on us. Multitasking was mandatory. Coffee breaks were not mandatory. We got to meet the local RCMP and were on a first-name basis with them in a very short time. Over the years, they would save us from many bad situations. We also helped them so it was a partnership from both sides.

After about two months I had to go back to Saskatchewan to write my RN examinations. So, after a busy set of shifts I was ready to see if I could pass the silly national exams that were made for people who didn't see blood and guts every day. I was never a bookworm. I was into getting my hands and my shoes bloody if needed and saving lives at any cost one at a time kind of person.

I had to drive to Saskatchewan after working a twelve-hour day shift. Another nurse named Donna wanted to come with me and I needed company to stay awake. After a twelve-hour shift, it was about a seven-hour drive. Donna was also working in the area and we had graduated together and got to know each other in our second year of school. We had an uneventful trip until we got to Saskatoon where we fueled up and grabbed a quick coffee. About half an hour down the road toward Davidson, we came across roadway construction: the highway was down to two lanes for several miles. After that, it became a four-lane again, but not for everyone. I noticed a car driving in the wrong direction heading southbound that was heading straight for the cars driving in the northbound lane. I was in the southbound lane. I had no phone and no way of getting help from the police. I wasn't sure what I could do but I wasn't going to sit by and watch them kill someone.

I told Donna that we needed to stop them. I reached under the seat and pulled out my red rotational light from my EMS days. We used it from time to time, even if it wasn't really legal. So, across the ditch I drove and the chase was on. I had a Ford Ranger that was built for speed. Donna said, "You can't do this," and I looked at her and said, "Just watch". It took me a bit to get the guy to stop but I did. I walked up to the driver's door and found exactly what I expected inside: one very drunk driver who should not have been driving with a sleeping passenger beside him. I thought to myself, now what? I still had no way to get ahold of the police. I wasn't sure what to do. At least I had stopped them. That was my only real plan. No one was dead and we had the vehicle off to the side of the highway. But we still were in the wrong lane on the shoulder of the highway, with cars coming directly at us.

I thought just maybe the passenger would be better off driving, so I woke him up. I talked to them both and I thought the passenger seemed okay to drive. At least he was more alert and didn't seem as drunk. So being a nice guy, I let them go and told them to be careful and warned them about drinking and driving again. We both crossed into the southbound lanes and took off. Immediately the car took off speeding, and I thought "Shit." I wasn't going to do anything more about it, as I'd already pushed the limits. We drove on for about twenty to thirty minutes when I started to see red and blue lights everywhere. We soon came across the car surrounded by police. I guess, unbeknownst to me, they had received complaints about the car and were looking for it. When they tried to stop it, the driver refused and that's when they took them out police style. They ran them off the road. They weren't going to let them kill someone that night.

It occurred to me that when the guys in the car saw the police lights flashing, they probably assumed it was me again and that's why they didn't bother to pull over—or they just didn't care because they were so drunk. I wished I could have done something differently when I stopped them the first time but I couldn't have. I pulled over in front of the red-and-blue lights lighting up the highway and walked over to the first police car. I introduced myself to the RCMP officer and told him what had happened and what I had to do to stop the car. The officer looked at me and said, "You did what?" So, I told him again. I said I used to be the manager of the Oxbow & Area Road Ambulance service and I still had my red light and this was an emergency. I'm sure he didn't know what to say to me. He took down my information and then went over to talk to the other officers and, to my surprise, they proceeded to charge both guys in the car. I drove off and made sure I never went over the speed limit as I had already been involved in one car chase that night, and that was enough for me.

I think I scared the crap out of Donna as she had never seen anything like that before. I hadn't told her about my past as an EMT. Looking back, I was lucky we didn't get killed trying to save others or arrested for trying to do the right thing. But I was determined not to let that car hit someone head-on and kill a family on the holidays. I could not have lived with myself for looking the other way. I had seen a car of drunken people hit an RCMP officer trying to stop it during a high-speed chase once. That is how Constable Doug Butler was killed on Oct 16, 1982. Constable Butler was an RCMP officer in Oxbow, Saskatchewan, and he was a good man. So, in hindsight regardless of any punishment I could have incurred, I would do the same thing again if the situation arose.

I was so happy to get to Regina and see some friends while I was there to do my RN exams. The exams were scheduled over two days. We had four exams to write and they were very stressful, but you couldn't really study for them. On the second day, I was seeing my friend Joanne for lunch and she brought her daughter with her. This was after my third exam, so I had one more exam after lunch and then was going back to Wetaskiwin. I was also scheduled to work the next day so it was going to be a short night but I was ready for it. I was used to burning the candle on many days in the past. Sleep wasn't always my friend, anyway, so it was okay with me.

The next day I met my friend Joanne. Joanne was an amazing lady with a cute little girl. We had met in first-year nursing classes and had always had a close bond. We planned to meet after my 3rd examination for lunch and catch up on our recent adventures. On the way back from lunch, we were driving on the ring road in Regina when we came across a multiple-vehicle accident in front of us. So, I stopped and made sure everyone was okay. A lady from a nearby apartment building had come over to make sure people were okay, as well. She told me she would call 911 and then she left. A few minutes later, I saw her coming back and she was attempting to cross the two busy lanes of traffic. I looked up and a car was heading straight at her as she was walking toward me in the opposite ditch. The driver was looking the other way, toward us, rubber-necking at the first accident and speeding along, oblivious to what was in front of her car. I had no time to say anything as it was already too late. Joanne and little Casandra saw her get hit and there was nothing I could do to stop it from happening.

The car hit her doing about fifty to seventy kilometres an hour. It hit her at a slight angle and her legs and hips went flying up in the air. The car was going fast enough that her head smashed into the windshield and then she just flopped like a rag doll over the top of the car. I was running full speed toward her before she even hit the ground. I thought she would be dead. She landed with a loud thud, face down on the pavement. It was not something you could ever forget. I kept seeing it over and over in slow motion for days. This day was getting worse by the second. I still had a stressful exam to write and it wasn't looking good right now. I thought "Why could I not have missed this?" and then I knew I was meant to be there so I just told my brain to shut up and I got to work. We had a life to save and if I failed my exams because of it then I simply failed. I had some practice at failing or learning the hard way you could say as well.

She wasn't breathing. I yelled, "Let's turn her over and get an airway!" My friend Joanne ran to my truck and grabbed my EMS belt as it had artificial airways in it. The middle-aged female driver who hit her came right over and said to just leave her. I said, "We're turning her," and she said to me, "I'm a doctor." I said, "Get out of the way—we're turning her over and getting her breathing." Some others on scene helped us log roll her and I got an OPA in her right away and got her breathing. She had a pulse, so we had something to work with. Within a minute, the first EMS unit was on scene and one of the staff knew me from my Oxbow days. He said, "Dale just keep working on the airway." They packaged her quickly and loaded her into the ambulance while I kept suctioning and maintaining the airway. In what seemed like seconds, we were off, lights-and-siren, to the trauma hospital. I was promoted to the airway person in a hurry and it was not open to debate.

My truck was still sitting there when the unit started off the scene with the siren screaming, and my friend was still standing there, as I never had the time to say anything to her. Joanne jumped into my truck and followed us to the Plains Health Centre shortly after and waited for me to come out the back doors. On our arrival at the hospital, a trauma team took over and my job was done. I had to write a statement for the city police and then I could leave. I was still shaking I'm sure. When I went out to the ambulance parking area, Joanne was waiting and poor Casandra was saying, "Lady hurt." I was so thankful we got her to the hospital alive. It must have been so scary for Casandra, as she was only three or four years old at the time and had watched it all from my truck, which was right between both accidents. Joanne was very supportive of me as I was a wreck and still in shock, too.

Joanne drove me to my last RN exam. It was a sad day, as we were both going different directions in our lives. Joanne was off to her new job and I had to go back to mine in Alberta. We had such a special friendship that it was a difficult goodbye. I gave her and Cassandra a huge hug and never even had time to cry. Then I walked into the school I had attended for the last two years for the last time. I was a little late and one of the proctors came and grabbed me as soon as I had sat down and said, "Come with me." I was sure I was screwed. How could I have gotten this far and lose it all now, I thought as I was marched out of the big room. I was late and I was going to get kicked out for helping to save a life I thought but somehow my guardian angels were on my side again today.

She walked me to the middle foyer where we had spent hours studying and socializing for the last two years. A few of the other proctors also sat down with me and fortunately I knew one of them. That made me feel a little better for some reason. I had never had her as a clinical instructor but I had heard great things about her from my fellow students. They told me Joanne had come to the school after the accident and told them what had happened. When they learned about the horrific accident they knew it wasn't my fault that I was late. The one instructor knew I was an EMT as well as an ambulance attendant, and she knew I had to do what I did no matter what. They bought me a coffee and sat me down and talked with me and actually showed me they too cared. They said they would keep everyone in the room until I was okay and ready to write the final examination and then I would be allowed to go in and write my exam. As long as the students were kept in the room, I was still okay, and they had made that possible. I still had a chance to pass my exam.

So, whether directly or indirectly, everyone involved that day helped me more than I can ever thank them. The fact that they came up with a plan to let me try and write the exam even if I had broken the rules. When I arrived late from such a very important exam showed me that nurses could always make the right decisions despite the strict rules we were obligated to follow in most circumstances. In about fifteen minutes I said, "Let's get this over with." I kept having flashbacks and it was not pretty. No amount of water would wash those images from my eyes for days to come. I can still hear the car hit her just like it was yesterday.

To this day, I will never remember the exam questions that were put in front of me. I kept seeing that poor lady flying through the air, then hitting the windshield, sometimes in slow motion, and other time at super-fast speeds. It was the strangest thing ever. Our brain is so complex. After the exam, I walked out and got Donna and we left for Alberta. Over our drive on the way home I told her what had happened, but it didn't seem quite real. The next several days were a blur and something in my head just blocked it out so I could go on. In a mere, several hours of arriving in Wetaskiwin, I was back on shift and thankfully the day and the rest of the week went by without incident.

Over the next several years my real education began and I realized I knew next to nothing. The more I learned, the more I had to learn; it was mind boggling. We were challenged daily by medical emergencies, trauma patients, cardiac arrest, assaults, and many small disasters or accidents that left their marks on all of us, emotionally and physically. We made the best out of a bad situation and went on.

We worked so hard most days and were soon able to predict probable outcomes from our past experiences. One tragic night the ER was crazy busy. I was called out a few blocks from the hospital for a shooting with my partner, and I should have been more worried but we didn't know what we were getting into but still I was not scared. We didn't carry portable radios or cell phones. So, if you needed help or backup, it wasn't always easy to get. We had a VHF radio in the unit and that was it for communication. On arrival, we pulled up and a younger lady came running out of a house and came directly toward us. You could see fear in her eyes and her voice had that urgency that woke up your brain in a hurry.

She said, "He's been shot." I looked around and the police had not arrived and we had no backup. I turned to my partner and said, "I'm going in to do what I can. If I don't come back out, don't come looking for me." I grabbed the trauma kit and went in and hoped the shooting was over. I found out after I got inside that the victim had shot himself in the head. He had shot four shots into the wall around his head but on the fifth shot he did not miss the most crucial part of his forehead. It was bad mess and with one look I knew we were in huge trouble in more ways than one.

His airway was poor and his breathing was ineffective with blood everywhere. A gun was still lying across his chest. I picked it up and set it aside to assess him quickly. Amazingly, he still had a good strong bounding pulse. Most times, we would ensure our patients had an optimal ABC before we did anything at all. I quickly checked him out and only found one small but terrible hole, and it was not a good place to be shot. Within seconds, there were multiple police at my side and I knew instantly they had my back and they secured the scene. They quickly searched the house to ensure it was not a murder or that we had not missed the fact we had an active shooter. I had also been to calls like this that had in the end turned out to be a murder and a staged suicide so you never could be too sure you were safe.

Looking back, it could have gone really bad for me in seconds if there had been more than one shooter. As it was, my police partners and I quickly loaded the victim on to the stretcher and inserted an OPA, attempting to bag him every five seconds as we headed out the door as fast as we could go.

We took him out of the house to our waiting unit. At the same time as I was working on his airway, suctioning it to clear of blood, attempting to ventilate him, and then we were off flying toward the hospital. It was called "scoop-and-run" for a reason: safety first, but also getting the patient to the closest hospital with extra hands was essential. We also needed a blood bank and an OR was always your primary goal in bad trauma calls. Only in this case, the victim was way past anything we could offer him locally. That night, I took the radio mic as I called the local ER and gave his approximate age, then said, "Shot once in the head—he's bubbling white and grey matter out." I then followed up with the obvious, "And that is not good."

Upon arrival at the ER, he was packaged up and sent to the closest trauma centre in a very short time. Sadly, we all knew the outcome. Another life had been lost to suicide. This affected so many people, even if people didn't want to talk about it. The only good thing about this night was somebody, or multiple people, could and would receive tissue and organ donations. Over the years, we saw so many suicides and were always left emotionally bereft and at a lack for words.

The hardest part was giving the news to the family and especially the spouses or significant others. Many were in complete shock. They would never be the same after going through this type of personal hell. Many would not or could not talk about it but you could see the pain in their eyes and the tears on their faces. I know that their hearts had been broken. Several of them would go on to take their lives, too.

I was so blessed in those early days to work with such amazing staff. The RNs, LPNs and NAs worked as a team on every shift. Very rarely do I remember a power struggle other than some interventions when a staff member was about to make a lethal or tragic mistake. This would be no one person's fault but a system of errors. I was one of these staff members one day, mere seconds away from killing someone when I figured it out. I looked back and realized I had been set up for failure and vowed to never make the same mistake again.

One fine Friday I didn't have to work nights and had nothing planned. I was busy most of the day and was ready for bed around supper time as I'd been up since late afternoon the day before. So, I had been up for about twenty-four hours with no sleep when my phone rang. I made the mistake of answering my phone. I was being ordered in to work a twelve-hour shift, as they were short-staffed. So, off I went not knowing at the time that it would turn out to be one long and scary night. About 2:00 a.m. I had an aspirin (ASA) overdose patient I was trying to save and he had taken a lethal amount. He wanted to die and I was about to wreck his day and save him.

The physician had ordered the appropriate antidote, which consisted of 40 mEq of Potassium Chloride in a 1000 mL bag of Normal Saline (NS), one ampule of dextrose which is equivalent to D50W, and ten units of regular insulin. Seeing as I was so tired and working without breaks, I had come to my breaking point. I mixed up my syringes. I almost gave the potassium chloride IV push instead of the dextrose. At the very last second, I stopped and said to myself something is wrong. I caught myself and made sure I was doing the right thing. I was kicking myself so hard after that near miss. I had come so close to making the patient's wishes a reality. He would have received the fire from hell in his arm down the IV line and then his heart would have locked up as the potent drug hit his myocardium tissues. Death would have been instant and nothing would reverse its effect. I was too close to making a mistake and I swore it would never happen again.

So, after that day I was never ordered in again. The two times they called me and I answered, I refused. Work is important, but if we cross the line and our work becomes unsafe, we pay the ultimate sacrifice. I would take my punishment for refusing orders, but I never was going to come that close to making a lethal error again if I could help it.

The best thing about Wetaskiwin General Hospital was the number of patients you got to meet. Every day was full of challenges; no two days were ever the same. We had so many cardiac arrests, near-death cases that our shifts were always interesting and full of learning moments. If you wanted to work hard, this was the hospital for you. If you wanted to be lazy, it was not. I would see many staff stay for a short time and leave for a variety of reasons, but at the end of the day the "lifers" stayed and worked hard no matter what came through that door.

Sadly, we saw many young patients, as well—many pediatric traumas that were mostly preventable. Some of the worst were the child abuse cases and the others I always hated were the Sudden Infant Death Syndrome (SIDS) cases. We were never sure if abuse or neglect played a role in the SIDS deaths, but it was something we all wondered about.

We commonly came across patients who were malnourished, and looking back, it was very common for kids to be having kids. The cases I will never forget are the shootings and stabbings, as well as the motor vehicle collisions were kids were not restrained and ejected from vehicles and came in as a trauma code or were dead on scene. The pediatric cases had a way of sneaking into your soul and ripping it apart without any warning. No one was immune.

Thankfully, we all had each others' back and we always made the next shift work. We had to, and would, make the bonds with our colleagues tighter and slowly we would rebuild our self-esteem. Tomorrow was a new day. We also had many good outcomes with very sick kids so it was never all bad. Sometimes kids would be lucky and miracles would happen despite the hell they went through. Kids will always have a special place in most nurses' hearts. Sick and dying kids would also break pieces out of our hearts over time.

The biggest newest change in my career was that Advanced Life Support (ALS) was finally a reality and when it was used were that lives were saved and suffering was lessened in many cases. The level of care and the team approach was so much more proficient and the results so much more visible then anything I'd seen in my past working in EMS. We would often take a cardiac arrest patient to be alive and stable for transport despite the initial event. I knew very soon I could and would learn many ALS procedures that would enable me to slowly expand my critical care and emergency skills. I had thought I was just coming to Alberta for a year and soon I realized I wasn't going home. I had so many learning opportunities ahead of me so why leave if being there was making me a better person, I thought.

The other part of my job working ER in the WGH was doing operating room (OR) on-call. I had no operating room training and it was a huge learning curve. Thankfully, we were always buddied with an experienced staff member who kept us out of trouble. It was not my favourite job just because it was so acute and things happened very fast. The scariest situations I remember were the STAT caesarian sections to get a baby in severe distress out or intervene when a delivery was not progressing. It was several minutes of stress followed by thirty minutes of clean-up on many cases. The gifted surgeons did the work; we just helped them be faster or more efficient.

We had four main surgeons and they were amazing. They all did emergency room on-call plus had a busy family practice, and they all did OR when they were needed on many day or night shifts. Several of them did elective surgery during the week, as well, so the OR was a happening place most days. They were gifted all-around physicians / surgeons, in my eyes. They were trained by the best before coming to Wetaskiwin and they presided over many complicated cases and worked very hard.

I did my required time in the OR and was thankful for it, as when I became a northern nurse I used that knowledge to help fix many personal disasters. I had the opportunity to witness many kinds of situations and could fix most myself if I had to, just from watching the gifted surgeons perform the operations time after time. The gynecology surgeon would have been especially proud of me years down the road when we needed a surgeon and couldn't bribe any to come to an isolated northern nursing station.

The situation I am talking about required me to repair an almost fourth degree tear from a precipitous delivery on a sixteen-year-old that almost tore her in half. It took me about two hours to repair it, but with some IV antibiotics and some time to recover, my patient was a happy new mom who could sit down without a very sore bottom. Dr. Ganguly would have smiled all day had he seen the job I did after watching him perform it several times in the OR. So even though I didn't love my OR shifts at the time, they later allowed me to save help people and to also help perform skills to save lives.

The one gentleman I have to talk about is Barry Wright. He was ex-military from the Canadian Forces and after retirement become a LPN. This is an amazing career change after spending twenty-five years serving his country all over the world. Barry was an excellent LPN who was known for driving the ambulance like it was a sports car. Barry could sure drive the unit and get us to the scene and back in record speed. Barry was on many serious calls with me. On our down time, we would share our own war stories. We both had stores but from different parts of the world.

There was one call that I will never forget that was a bad accident that happened just east of town. We staffed the ER with two staff in addition to responding to many ambulance calls, all while the night supervisor covered us in the busy ER. We arrived on scene to find one huge mess. Two trucks had collided at an intersection. There used to be a camper on one truck that had come off, and sadly the kids were sleeping in the camper when the accident occurred. The family had just been to the city and was shopping for groceries. I will never forget the groceries, especially the macaroni and the kids lying all over the highway.

One of the kids needed to get off scene faster than the rest. We grabbed the child who had been impaled in the side by a metal object and slid him into the back seat of an RCMP car and sent him off to the local ER. We then grabbed one girl, whose left side of her face had been peeled wide open, and sat her in the captain's chair in the back. This was not normal practice, but in a disaster, you made it work and we had to take everyone the first time around. We only had two stretcher spots and they were reserved for the severely injured parents on that call.

We knew how to look after trauma and tonight was the real test. Our education that night came directly from the trauma textbook we used, the *International Trauma Life Support* (ITLS) book. Back then it was a purely an American-based textbook and was used as our standard of care. It told us we had a golden hour to get everyone off the scene and to the hospital.

Looking back, we were on scene less than ten minutes, which is referred to the "platinum ten minutes;" the more time you spend on scene the higher the rate of mortality is with severe trauma patients. The biggest priority after you arrive on scene is to stop the bleeding or slow it down as much as possible, as soon as you find it.

We needed another ambulance but we didn't have one. We couldn't sit on scene and wait for more to come. So, we placed the broken parents on the only two spine boards we had and loaded them into the unit and were off in record time. On arrival, we had staff from all over the hospital pulled in to help, plus an extra doctor was called in. We were starting IV's, assessing, medicating and packaging them as best as we could. In two hours, we had them all stabilized. The X-rays, the preliminary lab work was done and out the ambulance door they went, off to the trauma centres that were on standby waiting for them. Miraculously, no one died that day. We saved them all with everyone working as a team.

We did the very best we could with minimal staff. This was before an air ambulance was available, but thankfully that night and on many other days, we had the city of Leduc sending us an ambulance as well as Muskwachees Ambulance Authority services (MAA). We used MAA many times for our critical care transfers over many years. They were a very good Advanced Life Support (ALS) service. We used the staff from MAA to transfer our patients that night as quickly as possible. There was a lot of blood lost, but in the end, we managed to slow the bleeding down and get it under control and we got them to the right place were the surgeons could do their magic with the blood bank right next door.

One of the hardest-working people I ever me was a man by the name of Marvin Hiller. Marvin was a LPN as well, and when we drove the ambulance, he was one of the best. Marvin had acquired a great work ethic from farming and when he came to work, he was a true caretaker. Marvin was always there if you needed someone to talk to and you could always count on him in times of need. The other staff that I worked with who made those days a lot of fun were Fran Greene, Rhonda, Wes Dorman, Dale Olson and Edie Ano. These people never let me down. It was a privilege to work with all of them for as long as I was able to.

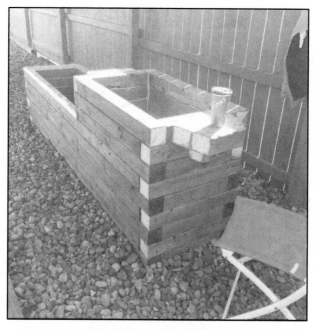

*"Building for the Future"*

*Chapter 8: Getting My Hands Bloody*

# "Risking It All for the Price of Life"

The real start in my medical knowledge came while I was in Wetaskiwin and a lot of it came within the first two years of being in Alberta. I had attended three amazing courses. The first was an Advanced Life Support (ACLS) course, then I took the Pediatric Advanced Life Support (PALS) course and finally I got into an Advanced Basic Trauma Life Support (BTLS) course. I also got in on a few smaller courses just to round out my knowledge even more in other areas. Few things in my life worked out as I thought they would but after a lot of personal effort, my dreams were becoming clearer. But the most valuable learning came from working with such dedicated people and from seeing the craziest cases. From shootings to car accidents, camper rollovers and farming accidents, cardiac arrests, child abuse cases and many severe beatings—I saw it all. I remember at least three separate homicides in the first year I was working at WGH and those were just the ones we couldn't save. There would have actually been many more deaths by homicide if it wasn't for the EMS crews, hospital staff and the quick and efficient system we had to get people seen quickly, stabilized and transferred out of our ER or to an OR quickly. It was truly mind-boggling to say the least.

One case I will never forget involved a young man who'd walked in front of a semi to end his life. His shoes were still on the road and he'd landed in the ditch. EMS scooped him up and brought him to us. On arrival, he was a mangled mess but still alive. The doctor was yelling at me to get a pelvis X-ray all while brain matter was coming out his nose. I said, "We have brain matter coming out his nose—maybe airway management or ventilation would be a better place to start." I remember the doctor yelling back at me, "He can lose two units of blood from his pelvis." But if you could have just seen the injuries. I knew that much more than two units were already on the floor and his estimate was a little low.

I remember him completely broken: bad airway, nasty chest injuries, his abdomen distended, and one side of his pelvis split wide open. The open side of the pelvis was broken off and rotated up into his abdomen cavity. This was the one of the worst cases I'd seen where the patient was still alive. His extremities were all broken and not easy to splint or manage but we got IV's in right away despite the fractures and they were running wide open. We grabbed four units of blood and a bunch of lactated ringers commonly known as RL. An ER doc jumped in the waiting unit and we took off for the trauma hospital. On arrival, we had already infused ten liters of IV fluid, four units of blood—and most of it was heading to the floor of the ambulance as soon as it could find a hole in the vascular bed someplace. My job for most of the trip was changing IV bags as fast as possible and I was also adding blood bags until they were all gone. I was constantly squeezing pressure infusers to push in the fluid and keep up to the heart rate, and we were losing it just as fast.

My hands were cramping as I was squeezing the inflation bulb so quickly and so hard. Talk about turning blood into Kool Aid especially in colour and a hemoglobin (Hgb) which would normally be in the range of about 120 g/L to 140 g/L before injury to around 30 g/L post our care. I heard he made it to the OR and that was that. He could not go on anymore. His poor body had been assaulted, beaten and time was never going to heal his injuries. When the semi drove into his body, he was already dead, but it took a few hours to declare the loss.

Still, we never quit trying to save him. He was someone's son, someone's brother and someone loved him. I just wish they could have watched the effort we were giving from the side lines. We had given all we had and, despite the odds, got him to the trauma centre alive. On the way back home, we stopped at a McDonalds for a burger and a drink. We were all exhausted and needed refreshment. I ordered a Big Mac and a soda. It was okay until I tried to eat it. In thirty seconds, I had completely wrecked my sandwich. Looking down, you could see my hands were still repeatedly squeezing or "bagging," and they had destroyed my Big Mac. Somedays you win and somedays you just lose.

The type of trauma that amazed me most was chest trauma. We once responded to a call from someone who had shot himself in the chest and was arguing with the nurse over the phone about shooting himself in the heart. She said," If you'd done that, you would be dead." He said again, "I shot myself in the heart" so we went to see for sure. We arrived on scene and found him with a hole in his chest and an exit wound in his back. He had missed his aorta by two millimeters, so technically they were both right. He was one very lucky man that day. Despite the bullet going right through his body, he was alive and was sent to a psychiatric unit for a sleepover after his required intensive care unit (ICU) stay with a chest tube to reinflate his collapsed lung.

What amazed me was how much blood someone could loose and still live. Then the next patient would have very little blood loss and die away. I got well versed in the injuries that are most likely to result in death. They are known as the "Deadly Dozen." The Deadly Dozen was also known as "the lethal six and the hidden six." The lethal six are airway obstruction, tension pneumothorax, cardiac tamponade, open pneumothorax, massive hemothorax, and flail chest, which are immediate threats to life. The hidden six are thoracic aortic disruption, tracheobronchial disruption, myocardial contusion, traumatic diaphragmatic tear, esophageal disruption, and pulmonary contusion. The last six are all serious events that can hopefully be found on the secondary survey but are commonly picked up in the computerized tomography examination as well as with ultrasound in the ER. They are easy to learn but a little harder to rule out in the pre-hospital care setting. Sometimes you treat for the worst and hope for the best; if a patient is meant to survive it will happen. The Deadly Dozen all require admittance to a specialty centre to assess, intervene and repair if possible. The only thing we can do is try to fix the airway obstruction, ASAP. We often tried to get our patients transferred very early even if any of the deadly dozen were expected and when working EMS all the situations happily met the trauma bypass protocols.

Tunnel vision always occurs if you're distracted by one problem and results in you missing the whole picture. You should always perform a complete and unobstructed assessment of the patient and try to spot the most common injures before the X-ray finds them for you. That is why a good doctor will stand back, usually at the patient's feet, where he or she can see everything, hear everything and be free to ask questions and clarify concerns as they are brought up.

While it is true that all of the Deadly Dozen chest injuries are life-threatening, often a patient will have other injures that we can't overlook. Over the years, we got better at sending out our trauma patients sooner to a trauma centre, but there is still a trend for some rural hospitals to hold on to patients for too long. By looking at the MOI, and by listening to the dispatch information from the initial call, you can initiate the normal trauma bypass protocols early. Then you will most likely get your patient to the trauma centre while there is still time to intervene. The biggest concern is always that we are missing the older patients who are dying or who have worse outcomes from even trivial injury, as we may initially diagnose these as trivial when they are actually not, due to the patient's age.

A simple serum lactate test scoring over two is indicative of severe internal injury. In places in the USA they are being done to initiate the trauma bypass protocol early and this helps save lives. STARS crews are actually using the fast scan on trauma patients and this is the newest wave in tools to quickly decide the most appropriate care and ensure quicker surgical intervention when required. When I say I got my hands bloody, I might have neglected or omitted to say there was also blood on my shirt, as well as my pants and very often all over my boots, as well.

Only once do I remember blood actually filling up on the inside of my one runners. This is possible if it runs down your arm and your foot or your leg was in the way. Blood or bleeding was never the scariest part for me, but when a patient ran out of it, it was very troubling, to say the least. We got used to giving lots of blood products fast without even thinking about protocols. In later years when tranexamic acid (TXA) was introduced, it would save more lives and we would have to use less blood products because of it. TXA is an amazing drug used to slow or stop bad bleeding that has saved many people in the short time it's been on the market.

I will never forget the nurses I started out working with and, looking back, I was blessed to have met some of the best staff imaginable. One of the greatest things about those early years was the excellent education system we had at our hospital. Joyce was the head of education and when she was in charge, and with the right administration, we had the best education system anywhere.

We had many adventures while working in the ER but one night I almost got my head taken off just for being in the wrong spot at the wrong time. That night I had been asked to work a twelve-hour shift as they were short an LPN. That was fine with me. It would be easier than normal as I would be buddied with an experienced

RN. As expected, the first part of the shift was a breeze. Around three in the morning, my coworker went for a break, and I was left by myself in the ER. I noticed a car drive into the ambulance bay and went to see what was up. There, I was greeted by a lady asking for help. I took one look and could see the trouble right in front of me. In the back seat of the car were three big kids and it looked as if a battle was already in progress.

One boy was being pinned down in the back seat by his two big brothers. They were on both sides of him and trying to keep him pinned down as hard as they could. I quickly ran to the nursing desk and grabbed the phone. I pushed the RCMP back-room number as it would get a quicker response than calling 911. A member answered and I said, "This is Dale from the hospital," while out of the corner of my eye I could see the boy coming straight at me. I just let the phone drop and then he hit me at a full run and never even slowed down. He went right over me and smashed my glasses into my face and took my watch off all at the same time. It was like being hit by a steamroller. Then I realized other people were in his path, and they were next.

To this day, I have no idea how I caught up with him but I had him in about five long strides and then I hit him like a bulldozer. He went crashing down to the floor and I was on him in a split second. I yelled at the people close by to go behind the desk and push the Code Blue button. They did and in seconds the Code Blue was ringing throughout the hospital. The first wave of backup arrived quickly and his two brothers also landed on top of me. His two brothers had joined the fight but they were on my side. I was holding him as tightly as possible in what amounted to a near-lethal chokehold, as nothing else would slow him down. He was lifting us all off the ground, which was more than 600 pounds if you added us all up. In seconds, more staff arrived and I yelled for them to stay back but get ready if we needed more help. I didn't want to hurt the kid, but I was so close to breaking his neck or choking him out and he was still fighting with the strength of ten men. I couldn't believe the strength. Then the real backup arrived.

With lightning speed, six big RCMP officers came running in through the emergency doors in tactical stance, with their guns out and ready to shoot. What they found was us fighting for our lives with the wall and floor already soaked in blood. They quickly took over and the boy was subdued and restrained. One of the officers helped me up and noticed the blood everywhere. One of the officers told me it looked as if he had been hit by a tree. All I could say back to him was "The tree was moving." And just like that it was over. My glasses were smashed and my watch was destroyed. I was a bloody mess but mostly intact. My nose needed sutures and I needed ten minutes to slow my heart rate to under 160 beats per minute (BPM). I still could not believe I caught him before he mowed the bystanders down like bowling pins. It was one day my speed was just right to win the race to save a life even if it meant me bleeding a little extra, it was worth it.

Over the next three hours, he remained in a crazed state and then he all of a sudden came back to normal. We found out he was doing PCP, which is also known as Angel Dust. Thank God nobody was seriously hurt that night. I was lucky I'm built like a John Deere tractor. But if he had hit one of the female bystanders standing at the triage desk, he could easily have killed them.

I think in that one year I was punched in the face about three separate times. It didn't really bother me or hurt, but I kept breaking my glasses. A few nights later one of the RCMP officers I met that crazy night was introducing me to one of the new recruits. He introduced me as Dale, then said, "When you need help, he just shows up." I didn't want to say I have a Radio Shack scanner and had nothing better to do when I was off shift most nights, but it was the truth. The first several years in the Wetaskiwin ER were never boring. Most people in our community probably had no idea of the many complex situations we had to deal with as nurses throughout the night while most of the city stayed in bed and had a good sleep. We had many violent or abusive patients that were normally nice people when they were not under the influence of alcohol or the wrong medications.

One of the strange parts of the job was the number of different types of cardiac arrests or Code Blues in our local hospital. The traumatic arrest was one of the main causes of a cardiac arrest that we commonly faced. We were able to get many of our cardiac arrest or "codes" back or help them in some way or form. But many of our Code Blues had tragic outcomes, as well. One day we had a traumatic arrest that was not turning out well and we were obviously losing the battle to save a life when a strange event happened that I just could not believe. The trauma arrest was in the trauma room and most of the patient's blood was on the floor or still at the scene of the original crime. No matter how hard we worked or how much epinephrine we gave the patient, we knew the outcome would be the same. Just before we called the code, a gentleman walked past the trauma door with a knife sticking out of his upper back. I told him we would be right with him. I realized it could be very serious, but seeing as he was walking I figured we had a few minutes. Then, a few minutes later, he walked the other direction past the trauma room doors all while reaching over his shoulder to his back. He pulled out the knife and looked at us, said "F--- you" and walked out. And that was that.

There wasn't much we could do about him, anyway. He had a knife, he was mad and we couldn't help him fast enough despite doing our best. I never saw or heard from that patient again. You've just got to do your best with the patients you have and the rest will look after itself on most days. All bleeding stops eventually so they say. If that guy really needed help, he would have passed out and we could have triaged him and gotten him into a room right away and fixed him up. But when you refuse to be triaged and walk away, we can't fix you. It wasn't his day to die. He likely had a few more lives left in him.

In the ER, we try to triage (assess and prioritize the most serious stuff) and treat the patients who need it most first. Sometimes I wonder what kind of lives these people must have to be involved in this type of violence day in and day out? It sure made me thankful to go home at the end of a shift and hang out with my golden retrievers, knowing they had my back. Sadly, many families see violence and abuse daily and it never truly stops.

Sometimes bad events can actually seem humorous after the fact. Someone might be in cardiac arrest and something so bizarre happens that it breaks the ice for days to come. Over the years we had many great nurses on the ER floor, but the ones that stood out to me most were the Licensed Practical Nurses (LPNs). In the early years, they were expected to be our drivers on ambulance calls as well as our partners in the ER on many lonely nights when it was just the two of you to take care of anything that happened. After we transferred to the new hospital site, the LPNs only worked in the ER as the new ALS service took over, putting an end to their driving days.

Over the years, I had the pleasure of working with Terry, who was secretly referred to as "Terrible Terry," by some staff who were afraid of him. Once you got to know him, though, you realized he was actually a very dedicated man who would never leave you stranded. He frequently went out of his way for patients, nurses and other staff. But you would not want to cross him—and, thankfully, I never did.

The funniest thing I ever saw Terry do was almost make a nursing student die of shock. We came in with my EMS partner with a real code from hell. It was an older gentleman who had gone into sudden cardiac arrest while driving his car and then his vehicle lost control and crashed after he had fallen unconscious at the wheel. The car then struck a set of gas pumps in Millet—at a lower speed but still scary—and there could easily have been a big fireball. My partner and I got the guy out of his car and put him into the unit. We had responded and ran the code by ourselves and a second unit helped us during the transport. It was a pure load and go call for two reasons: the scene wasn't exactly safe with the damage to the gas hazards, explosions risk, electrical risk of sparks and it was really cold out so we just loaded him up and started CPR in the unit. It's called an emergency evacuation and you back your unit away to a safe location with everyone still alive and intact. If the car had blown, we would have still been too close, thinking about it now. We could have been vaporized in a mere second.

It was most likely a medical event that caused the accident. Therefore, the likelihood of trauma-related injures was much less. One of us got the IV in and we followed it up with the first dose of epinephrine as he had a complete flat heart rate called asystole. Right after he went right into ventricular fibrillation so we immediately shocked him once. I was going to intubate him next, and that is when it went to right to hell. The feathers started coming, and they kept coming with each chest compression. I was knocking feathers from my field of vision as I readied the endotracheal tube, cursing the down-filled Arctic jacket he wore that had been compromised by a very sharp pair of scissors. You only made that mistake once in your career, then you took the jacket off every time and left your trauma shears on your belt. Every chest compression brought more of the goose-down feathers floating across the unit. We were off the scene in a flash, along with doing CPR all the way to the local ER while fighting off millions of feathers.

When the doors to the back of our unit opened in the ambulance bay, the feathers attacked everyone in the whole ER department and then followed us to the trauma room. The darn jacket was still under the man and still making it a feather war. Terry was in there like a dirty shirt for his role performing chest compressions. Terry was pushing hard and fast long before the Alberta Heart and Stroke Association or the American Heart Association (AHA) ever thought about making it a rule or the standard of care. The CPR was phenomenal. But then Terry started to sweat as he was working hard. The man in cardiac arrest had been stripped of all his clothes and a small facecloth draped over his groin, as was standard protocol. So at least we had stopped the continual feather attack.

Terry yelled at someone to wipe his forehead and his face to remove the excessive perspiration. The 495-senior nursing student that was buddied in the local ER never hesitated to get involved. She grabbed the facecloth and had almost touched Terry's face with it when he yelled, "Not that f---ing cloth!" Several of us laughed, but we weren't trying to be rude. It just broke the tension from the feather nightmare we had just come from. The gentleman actually ended up dying from a ruptured abdominal aortic aneurysm. So, no matter what we tried, the outcome would've been the same. He was still dead no matter how hard the CPR was that night. Despite the determined fate, we tried everything possible but it was in vain.

The poor nursing student immediately melted away and one of the senior ER nurses went to her side to make her feel a little better. I'm sure she had a bad night that night for it was such a traumatic event for many reasons: her first code, then it was such a mess, and then getting yelled at by Terrible Terry. Terry apologized to her and you could tell in his heart he was not trying to be mean; it was just who he was. I respected him greatly and got to be good friends with him for years—so good, in fact, that I asked him to be the best man at my wedding. To anyone that knew Terry he was a gentle sole but could be heard from the dead.

Over the next number of years in WGH, I grew more and grew in my knowledge and skills. With every shift, I learned something new. I saw pain like none other on some calls but few; I also saw love and pure dedication from people who truly cared about everyone they touched. If I could, I would do it all again, and I wouldn't change a thing.

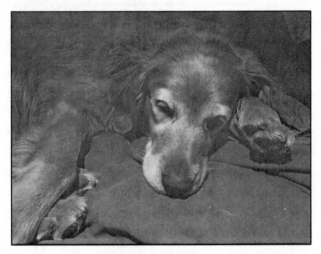

*"Wisdom from Within"*

## Dale's 10 Trauma Rules to Remember

1. *Gunshots to the face and head are bad.*

2. *Chest penetration is bad, especially in the area of the heart and greater vessels.*

3. *Brain matter on the floor is bad.*

4. *Stab wounds to the neck are not good.*

5. *Sucking chest injuries are bad.*

6. *Stab wounds to the abdomen are never straightforward.*

7. *Missing arms and legs are not good.*

8. *More lacerations or fractures then you can count on one hand is bad.*

9. *You can't defeat the Law of Physics.*

10. *Stupid people have the right to die from their own stupidity, but not from yours.*

# "Real Nursing"

My biggest adventure in nursing started north of the 60th parallel. I liked the challenge that working at a northern nursing station offered me. Nearly all of the stations were located on the First Nations reserves and you were it, as there was no backup. You had no one to help you and you had to handle anything that came along until a medevac plane arrived and could get help to you in these most isolated of locations.

My first several postings were excellent. I had very experienced staff who helped me with the process and made good decisions. In the more complex cases, we could always phone a physician. We would see lacerations, which we would suture up, provide immunization boosters, provide wellness clinics and see to sick walk-in patients. The hardest cases were the kids and the odd woman in labour—those always made our heart skip a beat.

With pregnant women, if at all possible, we got them sent out two to four weeks before their delivery date as weather—especially during the winter season—was so unpredictable. We got good at measuring fundal height, auscultating fetal heart sounds, and we were always happy when the plane or ambulance had safely taken off with mom-to-be inside. Over the years, I worked at six separate stations up north and had stories that would shock most people from each one of them.

One of the worst cases I attended to was a drowning at a church retreat. Two young girls had been playing by the river when they suddenly disappeared. We feared the worst. We went right away to help but, tragically, it was too late. Upon our arrival, the first girl had already been located by her family and friends. She drowned in warm water and it was too late to try to perform any heroics as it would be of no benefit for anyone. We ended up transporting her back to the station. It wasn't until the next day that the second girl was located by the RCMP divers who'd arrived on the scene right after we did. Their job really must suck some days. They see the worst of the worst and go from one bad disaster to the next and then they are expected to go home and act like everything is okay. I'm sure they'd just go home and hold their kids tightly and cry themselves to sleep some nights.

That incident showed me how strong people could be and how they came together in times of trouble and made everyone part of the family. After that day, the people of the community respected us even more and we were more accepted into their community, even if there was little we could have done for the girls. We helped transport the second dead girl to the coroner to get her ready for the funeral that was to come. After that day, I never wanted to see another downing victim for as long as I lived, but I would, anyway, in the ensuing years.

One day we had a gentleman who wanted to shoot himself sitting on a quad with a gun right outside our buildings. I thought, "Well, this could go one of two ways. Either he shoots me or he shoots himself." The smartest plan was to wait at the nursing station until I heard a bang or until the RCMP arrived. A short while later, the quad started up and he was off to somewhere else. The police later came and arrested him and that situation was uneventful. When he was ready to be flown out I ensured he was sedated enough to not be a problem in flight. I had ensured my pharmacology calculations of just the right combinations of medications maintained a zero chance of anyone being hurt in flight.

I always felt bad for the police. More often than not, their presence was unwelcomed and they were frequently hated for doing their job. They would rely on us for backup and we relied on them even more when we had trouble or needed help. I remember even making them a homemade meal when they got stuck in our community, waiting for additional backup. It was a northern thing we just did. We were always a team. They needed us but we needed their presence even more.

We travelled the local community in Chevy suburban 4x4s or Ford Explorers. Sometimes we picked up sick people and brought them to the stations; we also used them to set out the landing lights at night for the medevac planes. Our Community Health Reps (CHRs) also used them to visit with people in the community. One day I came across an injured horse. I thought it was just sick and would or could use some IV therapy to help it out. This wasn't on my list of skills, but in a pinch we looked after sick animals as veterinarians didn't exist in these remote locations. I checked out the horse but could not figure what was wrong right away. It looked to be in shock. I was going to treat it with IV solution and do anything possible if needed but I would not have enough IV solution to matter. So, I decided to flip the horse onto its other side and there was the problem. The local dogs had chewed a big hole in its hind quarter. They had eaten part of the horse and it was still alive. It was so tragic. The poor horse was never going to make it. There was no magic remedy I could give it. It made my heart sick.

I went to the closest house and knocked on the door and when it opened I asked for a gun. They said, "No gun," which I guess was the right answer. I then looked at one of the elders and said to one of them looking at me from the front door that I needed a gun to shoot a horse. The younger man was then approved by the elder to help and then he reached behind the door where I was standing and passed me a loaded rifle. I reluctantly went and shot the horse. I couldn't fix it, but I could make it so the horse didn't have to suffer. It was not my normal job but it was part of the role as a northern nurse if you could stomach it. We were not always a nurse.

Back in my childhood, I had to do the same thing and often to horses worth thousands of dollars. Some were our best friends but it didn't matter; it was still the right thing to do even if it hurt doing it. I took the rifle back to the owner, minus one bullet, and drove away knowing it was a terrible waste of a good horse. Somethings you can't fix or change and this was one of the things. All I could do was put the horse down and end his suffering. The dogs would be back soon enough but I could not stop that from occurring.

The northern nursing stations had the coolest people in the whole world. The nursing stations I worked at included Fox Lake, John D'Or Prairie, Assumption, Atikameg, and Fort Chipewyan. The people were all different and the communities all had their unique, good, and some not so good, parts. I loved Fox Lake as the people were so nice even if they were not as educated as in some of the other places. The ones that intrigue me the most were the people from Fort Chipewyan, though, as they had such a different land presentation, which in pictures reminded me of parts of northern Ontario I'd seen in books. The people I worked with there were educated and much more advanced than the other isolated communities. Every one of these communities was unique; they each had their own heritage and pride, and I know if given the chance they will do great things.

Fox Lake was a big eye-opener for me as we never had two days the same. One of the most memorable events was assisting in a delivery with another nurse, who to this day I must say was the best of the best. Chris Ryan was the acting charge nurse and came from the east coast. He was so calm and cool no matter what came through the door. Well, this night a young lady walked in and she was too young to have a baby, but she was in active labour, anyway. I don't remember ever having seen anyone about to have a baby act so calm. She was smiling from ear to ear.

In minutes, we were in the middle of a bad delivery as she was just over forty weeks and the head was huge. It became stuck, with the shoulders locked in the worst place. We had no extra help so a caesarean or any form of assisted delivery was not an option. It was just me and my hands doing the delivery. Sometimes kids are born in just a few good contractions. But this was a much smaller, younger mum than normal, and it was her first delivery, as well. Plus, the unborn child's head was huge, which told me we were in deep trouble.

The labour had stopped progressing as the head was now stuck in the birth canal. In this position, the little guy was doomed. I grabbed a pair of sterile scissors and went to perform a midline episiotomy to try and make some room to get the newborns head out, and the flipping screw was part way out of the scissors. I didn't have time to run and get anything else; I was committed. I just kept making little tiny incisions by holding the scissors just so and slowly I got the job done. I quickly maneuvered the head and shoulders in just the right position and out slid an 8.5-pound crying baby. I was so relieved with Chris at my side, couching both me and the mum at the same time. We just about never had a success story like this, as delivery was so hard and when it stopped progressing it was rare to have a successful outcome. Today it was a good outcome despite the complications.

The whole time the poor mum was as silent as anyone I'd ever seen. An amazing, tough little lady she was. I'd seen multiple deliveries in other hospitals and I knew it sometimes got very loud, but that was not the case tonight. I took the pair of scissors and tossed them into the closest garbage so they could never get put in an emergency delivery bundle again. We had won the battle again and in no time had the mess cleaned up. The placenta was out and Mum and baby were doing well. Some Vitamin K for the baby, and antibiotic ointment for the little one's eyes and we were ready for a well-deserved coffee.

Sometimes you know you're in over your head and one day I had this happen out of the blue and all we could do was our best. A little child was brought in with a significant past medical history. On his record, it listed his conditions and also said that we would be unable to intubate him or perform a surgical airway due to abnormal airway structures. Well, this little one was very sick and the outcome appeared grim.

If you can establish an airway and get a patient breathing adequately, circulation will look after itself as long as it is not stopped. If you're not sure about life signs, it's best to just start CPR and then say a little prayer. One or both of these problems can result in cardiovascular compromise. We had a little memory tool we used for kids: A+B=C, which amounts to Airway + Breathing = Circulation. Whereas in adults, the formula is actually C=A+B, which essentially says that if they have circulation it most commonly eliminates the need for fixing the airway and breathing, and this also follows our new CPR approach for any unconscious patient. It's so much easier if you can just simplify things right away.

Often times we were presented with a sick child with a breathing complication on scene and learned this through his SAMPLE history. The more complex the SAMPLE history, the more impossible it would be to stabilize the patient, especially in the middle of nowhere. SAMPLE is an acronym for Symptoms, Allergies, Medications, Past Medical history, Last Meal, and Events leading up to the event or situation. We always just started with the simple stuff. We would apply the oxygen, suction the airway, clear the nose of secretions as needed and call for a priority medevac. Commonly, the patient would be suffering from a severe respiratory infection such as RSV or, worse, pneumonia. We were so pleased when the flight crew would arrive, package the patient safely and take the little person away to a better place. Our collective BP would drop by 20 per cent, I'm sure. Then it would be time for a coffee before heading back to work.

The majority of cases we dealt with were trivial and didn't take much to manage. But others were much more complicated. Patients might come in sick with small or vague complaints. Then quickly, you would realize the patient was septic, dehydrated and in acute renal failure. To top it off their blood sugars were greater than on any past visits. That was when you knew your day just got a lot more complicated. But your patient's day was always much worse. Early intervention could make a world of difference and if you sent them home, there was always the possibility they wouldn't make it.

The very best thing about working at the nursing stations was the dedication of the staff to their community. All of the staff but one person I met were amazing and the care they provided was first-rate. This one staff member had a problem with me being Caucasian, but it was the only prejudice I ever encountered, and it wasn't even from a patient. It was the 1st and last time at this one community I was thinking at the start of my 1st shift.

When hate is in the air, it can make it very difficult to keep working, especially when the prejudice is so evident. After five long days of working under these conditions that were completely due to this one particular staff member, I packed my bags and would never return to that location. I could understand patients hating Caucasians for the ineffective care they'd received in the past. But when you're in their place as a guest, and you're not wanted, it gets complicated right away. Thankfully, at the rest of the stations I repeatedly ran into wonderful people and the patients I had the privilege of helping formed a trust bond with me in no time. To this day, I keep in touch with some of them and they still call and turn to me for help when they need it the most. It is such a good feeling to know you have helped them in some of their most troubled times.

# "Amazing People"

The North had always intrigued me as a kid: *Mad Trapper of Rat River* was a good book I had read in elementary school and the Stompin' Tom Connors song, "Lost" always gave me goosebumps. The opportunity to work in Fort McPherson, NWT, as a community health nurse was so interesting to me. This would get me up to the real north, and it was a once-in-a-lifetime adventure. Even better, I'd get paid for the trip.

I could see and feel the true north as it still was despite the influence of the modern world south of it. When we arrived, I met the challenge to learn the culture and experience the northern traditions. In September 1993, we headed north as a family for an adventure and a lifetime of memories. My son was just a year old then and my wife had taken the year off from nursing to make the trip. The year wasn't as much fun for her as it was for me, and even though she may have hated me for it, I believe she had some good memories from the time, as well.

The drive was 3100 kilometres and was going to take three long days. We would need to drive from Wetaskiwin to Grand Prairie and then head into the northern part of BC. From there we would drive into the Yukon to the famous Dawson City, which was the home of the Klondike Gold Rush from another song when we were kids, Johnny Horton's "North to Alaska." We would then need a full tank of gas and to make sure the road was open, before the ferry would take us across the Peel River—if the ferry was ready and running—where we could start to head north up the Dempster Highway (a.k.a. the Yukon Highway). Finally, we would drive into the Northwest Territories. The road was going to be tough, rough and the weather would be unpredictable at best.

Before the trip, I did some research into a good 4x4 and we found an indestructible vehicle that met our needs. We purchased a 1990 Jeep Cherokee that was made for a northern adventure and off we went. The drive was without adventure until we arrived in Dawson City. The Dempster Highway is a gravel road that leaves civilization and heads about 425 kilometres in a northeasterly direction until you arrive to Inuvik, NWT. That is where the real road stops. Sometimes it is impassable and sometimes the ferry doesn't run due to freeze-up. Therefore, you need to always plan your trip well. That we had done: we had extra gas, a spare tire, food and drinks, and we thought we were ready. We had already taken one extra day, and after the three-day drive of paved road we were at Dawson City and we met the snow. Snow and cold meant that winter was coming much faster than expected. But the North has its own agenda with a unique schedule from Mother Nature. Our northern adventure was about to begin.

On that first morning travelling the Dempster, we started up the road and only got about forty kilometres before we had a flat tire on our driver's rear tire. We were loaded extra heavy and there was no shoulder or place to pull off the road, so I just had to stop and try to change the tire on the northbound lane. No big deal, I thought and got the car jacked up carefully with everyone staying out of the snow and cold while I worked fast and I tried to change it. Well, I couldn't get a few of the nuts off. Apparently when they put the tires on for us before the trip, they overtightened the nuts. I tried and tried but I could not break the nuts free. I'm a big strong man and had a really good tire tool, but it didn't help.

We sat for a few hours until a very nice transport truck driver came along and helped me. It took an eight-foot snipe to get them off. I didn't feel so bad after that about being weak. But we had wasted too much time and we could not be sure we would make it before the ferry shut down for the night, plus we had no spare tire. We turned around and went back to get our tire fixed and spent an extra night at a bed and breakfast. We planned to make the trip again as soon as first light was upon us. This time we made the trip without incident. My son didn't mind at all, as he was having an adventure of a lifetime. Plus, he got to learn to pee in the snow, which was good training for the future.

The drive was truly amazing and so uplifting. We drove past the tree line, which is where trees forget to grow very tall and remain little stubs, catching the snow. Then we went through the Richardson Mountains where the legendary North-West Mounted Police were lost and died from starvation and freezing to death. It's the one trip everyone who calls themselves Canadian should do to appreciate the True North. We didn't see many other vehicles, but everyone we met waved at us, which was not so common anymore back down south.

If someone was stopped or stuck along the way, it was customary to help no matter who it was or why they were stopped. You just stopped and helped them and they would help you in return if you needed it. You always had a tow rope or a chain handy. Money was not expected or transferred. The view out the car window was endless beauty as far as the sky went with no two pictures being the same. We stopped in Eagle Plains for a break, for more fuel just in case, had a great home-cooked lunch and an amazing, but slightly expensive, meal. That was the North. You never complained as it was food, and your options were limited to usually one place. Even in 1993, a bottle of Coke could cost you up to $3.00 during breakup and freeze-up so if you wanted it, you just paid your dues and enjoyed it.

The final leg of our drive was just as good and as soon as we got to Peel River and could see tents along the river's edge with smoke coming out of the chimneys, we were happy. The fishing camps were a good welcome sign and we knew we were almost at our new home. When we arrived, we were greeted warmly by all the station staff and right away we felt at home.

The first month was a big learning curve. We were so busy, plus I had to go to Inuvik for extra training. The CHR staff was amazing and made a point of making us feel welcome and part of the community. Mary and Whinny were the best community role models and leaders I would ever meet. They would interpret the local language, which was Gwich'in, from the elders and help us with local customs. Our life in the community was so much easier with them at our side or just a phone call away.

The local RCMP were also fantastic. Fort McPherson had an up to five-member detachment, and we soon got to know them all and would see them at all hours for help. Occasionally, we helped them out, as well. The leader was one of the best I've ever met. Staff Sargent Dales Erikson was the kindest RCMP officer I've had the good fortune of knowing and a true gentleman at heart. Over the next year, I'd see him in action several times and he was someone who could look after himself very easily. Then there was Howie Eaton as the senior corporal, as well as John Comier and Dave Wilkinson, whom I actually helped rescue in a wicked battle to live one day months later. Finally, there was Ron who was a very quiet but effective member. Northern policing was so much different than policing in the rest of Canada, as you were really just peacemakers and community therapists on the side.

We had a few nurses who were not so nice to the RCMP for stupid reasons and they didn't last long in the community. We would get some nurses who were very good and others who were not so good. A few were insane, but they earned a salary just the same.

These were the people you counted on throughout the long, cold winter, as well as the days of endless sun in the summer. The best northern nurse I have ever met was Elna Eidsvik. She was an ambassador for humanity, but at the same time she called it the way it was. Elna would attack any project and had the ability to simplify the complex problems and come out with a solution. Elna taught me that doing what was right for the patient was more important than to following protocol. Common sense would win in a difficult decision every time. I sure wished I would have known her my whole life as I would be much wiser and would have made the right decisions much quicker in many situations in the past.

Our shopping was limited to the Northern Store and the local co-op store. It had everything we needed, but at a cost. You went and bought what you needed and paid the price. Expiry dates were suggestions and not absolute as sometimes it was that or nothing. All in all, I never thought much about it. You watched your budget and you were more grateful then many are with a Walmart or McDonalds next door.

I soon realized the people from Fort McPherson were so much different than anyone I'd ever worked with or been around my whole life. They were much happier people, stronger people—much more grateful for everything around them and, most important, very proud people. I heard the stories of the Mad Trapper from families that had known him and knew the people who had helped catch him. They also told me the stories of the Lost Patrol and some people actually remembered Martin Hartwell, the legendary bush pilot. They were proud to be who they were.

I would learn of the people hunting on the land or hanging out along the Peel at the fishing camps for days. They were the proud people who still fished when the season was right and also some of the same few people who still used dog sleds to travel, even today. I would see skidoos used for their original purpose and I would see the snow so cold that you could drive your truck on it with no problems at all. Sadly, I would also see the effects of alcohol and abuse related to its effects all too often. This was a common problem for the police as well. We would also see the scary effects of chest infections, respiratory tract infections, cancer and sexually transmitted diseases. All in all, these were tough people and they were fighters to the end.

I was very privileged to be taken out hunting and to see the massive herd of caribou that would cross the Dempster for days at a time. If you have seen the movie, *The Polar Express,* it will transport you there, as well. As Tom Hanks says in this movie, "Sometimes the most real things in the world are the things we can't see." Well, believe me, it is one of the wonders of the earth, compliments of Mother Nature.

We responded to accidents, we did sick clinic most mornings, then in the afternoon we performed specialty clinics. These were geared toward the elderly, children and maternal health. We also offered immunization clinics. We even got to respond to emergencies along the Dempster Highway from Eagle Plains all the way to the Arctic Red River, which became Tsiigehtchic sometime in 1994. We also did a day clinic in Arctic Red River once a week, which was fun. The rest of the week it was looked after by a CHR on call or the patients got care in Inuvik. We had many interesting calls on the Dempster Highway over my year. I had the misfortune of coming across an unfortunate man who had crashed his mountain bike after riding down a hill and hitting a barrier. This was okay for me as I was a little seasoned by then, but it terrified the other nurses, as they were not into blood and guts. I'd had blood on my hands many times before this adventure ended.

One of the most memorable cases from me was when I had started to look after an elder who had become ill. We initially thought he just had a virus, but in time we found out he had terminal cancer.

There was a language barrier; I couldn't speak his language and he couldn't speak mine. But I could communicate with him at a deeper level with my use of touch. Therapeutic touch from someone with a caring heart can cross many barriers. I held his hand and found I was helpless to make his suffering go away.

The best I could do was by seeking help from people much wiser than I was. I was so lucky to be able to seek frequent knowledge and guidance from our always available Inuvik physicians. I was so naive to the use of medications for pain control that I ended up prescribing the highest dose of hydromorphone (Dilaudid) that I could imagine. The dosage I was administering could have easily have killed anyone in the wrong hands. In many cases, even one pill could kill someone—especially a child. In this case, it seemed to give him a break from the severe pain he was experiencing from the metastatic spreading cancer. I consulted our on-call doctors and we added extra classifications of medications that helped, but none seemed as effective as they needed to be. Sadly, we only took the edge off of his pain but he always smiled and was so thankful for everything we tried to help him. One sad day he just went to sleep for the last time.

Then I learned something I would not have ever even considered before. After his death, the community, being his family and friends, started to dig his grave. It took five days of digging in the cold and through the permafrost that was like cement. It was dug by hand and not by machine. It was dug with pride and love. I was so thankful for the privilege of being able to share in this valuable cultural event. To this day, he will be one of the toughest and strongest men I have had the privilege of knowing during his last battle to live.

The other amazing friendships that I forged were with the local RCMP officers. They were not as accepted by the community as we nurses were, but they were still appreciated nonetheless. Over time we got to share our lives with them and help them in times of trouble, as well. The coffee pot was always on and we were always treated like family every time we crossed paths in our travels.

I often made home visits to see their sick children, and suture rowdy or drunken prisoners who had been cut or stabbed in domestic altercations. I even performed plastic surgery in the jail on someone who needed some repair work before being taken to the territorial correctional jail. This was after I found him a healthy dose of medication for a treatable but nasty sexually transmitted disease and the mess I repaired on his face. I did some research and found an antibiotic that would work for both problems but made his backside sore for several days. It is amazing how effective antibiotics can be when used the right way, in the right doses and for the right reasons. Pillows can be used for a lot more than something to rest your head on in a hard, cold jail cell, I reckon, when you've just received two larger than normal injections in the backside.

The guy was very pleasant to me and I was not in any danger but I had a nice police officer at my side just the same. You got to feel comfortable with any situation when the patients or prisoners knew you weren't judging them but just trying to help them in their time of need. The officer in arm's reach was just a friend who was not leaving your side. It amazed me how comfortable the police had made me feel minutes after meeting them. Over time we got to having regular coffee dates, share stories and letting each other know we were one big family. They needed us but we needed them more. Then one day, I knew our friendship was for life.

On one memorable day Dave had stopped for coffee, and we chatted about the many things we had in common. Dave had vast experience as a police officer and had spent a little time in EMS, and once we started talking time went fast. Before long he had to go back to patrolling the community. I would listen to the police calls, fire calls and air traffic control from time to time so I would also listen to Dave as he travelled around the community as a solo member. I had a cool scanner and over the years I had used it a few times to respond to EMS calls before we were even dispatched, or to fire calls and even to help a police officer in trouble after he called a 10-33, which I knew to mean "officer in trouble" in the past.

A few hours later I heard my old reliable scanner clicking. I could hear what sounded like a radio trying to connect with the phone system. I looked at the frequency that was making the noise. It was the local RCMP frequency. I knew Dave was on patrol today on his own, which was common but also dangerous. So, I called him and took my chances of just making a silly call for nothing. Dave answered and what I heard was scary. "Dale, I need help," he yelled. He named his location and I was gone in a flash to get help. I grabbed the keys for our van, jumped in and took off for the RCMP compound to grab some reinforcements.

I pulled into the RCMP compound driveway and hit the brakes hard. I was out of the van before it stopped. I got out and yelled to whoever was listening, "I need a cop" and "I need a gun!" This was not a normal way to get help and, thinking back, it was almost crazy. I would never be disrespectful to the police, but I needed help and I had no time to debate the issue. Thankfully, in a few seconds John came running out of his house at full tilt and had a gun in hand that he was putting on his gun belt. In seconds, we were off. No questions and no explanation were needed or given just yet. I had backup now, and getting to Dave was my only concern. Dave hold on I was thinking as we are coming and we have firepower and we won't let you down. It would be my promise even if it was never stated.

I told John the situation as the tires were spinning out of the compound and he gave me the best directions. I drove as fast as possible and took the corners a lot faster than usual. I was driving tactical in a 4x4 minivan. We arrived to find a police truck in the driveway and no Dave. This was not a good sign. Where was Dave and, more important, was he okay? We knew nothing about the situation. The only place he should have been right then was inside the house in front of us. We had no idea of what to expect nor could we wait or call for backup. Dave's life was on the line.

Well, this wasn't my first tactical experience but I was unarmed and I had no vest, so bullets and knives would not have been good for my inner parts. Fortunately for me I was built like a tank so I could stop some metal without making myself dead as long it was not a large caliber bullet I had a fighting chance. We just moved forward as one, having no idea what lay ahead of us. John nailed the door at a dead run and I was right behind him. We found Dave right away and, just as expected, he was in big trouble. He was in the fight for his life. He just couldn't get the man down and he couldn't get his gun out to end the fight or to simply shoot him. No one wants to use their gun if they don't have to. Not one RCMP member I ever met had a desire to draw their gun unless the situation absolutely called for it. When it was kill, or be killed then they were taught they had no choice. Lethal force was something they were all taught to use but most reluctant to unless there were no other options.

We hit Dave's assailant hard and fast, not to hurt him but to win the fight. We had him down on the ground in seconds and the fight was over. I'm sure Dave could have kissed us both that day for saving his life. Dave got himself back together in a few minutes and quickly caught his breath. His body still needed a bit longer to recover from the side effects of adrenalin rush I was sure. While he rested, his assailant was handcuffed and put in the back of the police truck. Sadly, the whole event was often entirely fueled by alcohol use or abuse. Thank God Dave was okay and no one had to die that day. That day made our friendship even more special.

I was glad my Radio Shack scanner was on because it saved a life that day. Today I was much more than a northern nurse.

Not long after that incident, I decided to try and do something just plain crazy. I was going to hitchhike from Fort McPherson to White Horse in the Yukon to meet my wife. I had never done it before nor I have I done it since. My wife had drove home to Wetaskiwin for a holiday and after her break was then driving with my son Jonathon (JD) back as far as White Horse, Yukon. She was reluctant to drive the Dempster on her own with JD without help. So, I said, "Why don't I meet you and help with the long drive?" I had never hitchhiked in my life, but I knew the people of the North would look after me regardless of my reasons for making the sixteen-hour car ride with strangers. You could not find better, kinder and safer people to be with in the whole world. As long as alcohol was not involved, you were safe and free from harm. I initially got a ride to the Peel River ferry crossing, and there I waited. I was a new hitchhiker and I only had about 1500 kilometres left on my adventure. I had no idea my trip was going to be interrupted due to a real-life emergency.

When I was waiting at the ferry I figured I would ask people if they were heading south and I knew in my heart that it was okay and I was never in any danger. I asked a few people but they said no. Then I was asked to come over to a northbound truck by the ferry captain who knew I was also the local nurse. The driver of the truck had stopped somewhere along the Dempster when he had found a man injured after a mountain bike accident. He was lying in the back of the truck and he looked hurt and was also a bloody mess. But he was still smiling. This smiling man was very nice even if his English was not his first language, but he was a fit tourist visiting from another country and he was now my patient. I'm sure when he went down the steep hill he never dreamed trouble was coming just before he lost control and crashed his bike into a safety rail. He was planning to ride across the whole

North over the summer and then fly back to his home country. I never expected this, but sometimes life happens for a reason.

All I remember vividly was his nasty open neck injury. He had hit a guardrail, which was most likely why his poor neck was cut wide open, plus he had other injuries, but the mess to his neck made me worried. The carotid arteries were visible, pulsating and just so vascular it would be tricky and difficult to fix even for a surgeon. I'd done some pretty good suturing but I knew in an instant this was way out of my league. So, I jumped in and that day I was a paramedic again. I applied direct pressure to the side of his neck, but not hard enough to cause bad cerebral perfusion, and we made a speedy trip to the local nursing station was about all I could do for him. The helpful family in the truck that found him took us back to Fort McPherson and my holiday was delayed just a bit more. But this was why I lived and breathed and I would not complain a bit. On many occasions, I was either unlucky or lucky to be in the right place at just the right time.

On arrival, the nurses were shocked to see me, as one of them had left me at the ferry crossing a few hours before and we had planned to have coffee in three days when I came back so I could share my hitchhiking story. Well, the story so far was short and bloody, you might say. I remember the look in her eyes. But she was even more shocked to see this man and his significant neck injuries. We immediately inserted some big IVs into him, all while treating him for shock with warm blankets and getting him to lie supine. They had called for a medevac plane that was inbound as soon as possible. After he was stabilized, one my friends from the RCMP offered to take me back to the ferry to try one more time, and just like that I was a hitchhiker all over again. It was rather odd getting a ride to the ferry with the police to then hitchhike but again this was the north and it had its own rules and its own customs.

Back at the ferry, I said thanks to my police friend for the lift and then I tried a few more times to get a ride. Soon, a small station wagon belonging to a nice family from Inuvik came onto the ferry. I asked if they had room and could I get a ride. They said they would but they were too full. I said no trouble and that was that. They got on the ferry and rode across. I thought I was going to strike out and that my hitchhiking days were over before they got started when the station wagon drove off from the ferry, pulled over and stopped. The male driver got out and called to me, "Get in!" They squeezed over and I was off to meet my family with one of the nicest families I have ever met.

They treated me like royalty. The kids made me enough room even though the back seat was already full. We started talking and I could not believe they also knew my uncle's nephew in Inuvik, who was from Carnduff, Saskatchewan, my home town. That just amazed me. It made me realize and, even more, showed me the world is even smaller than we all think. In no time, we arrived in Dawson City, and they found some food for the road for themselves and also for me and we all grabbed some drinks. Then we got some lifesaving gasoline, had a spare tire fixed and we were off. They would not take money for the trip, for the food, or for the gas. They shared what they had with me and gave me all the food I could eat and expected nothing in return. They refused to take money from me. After they dropped me off, I got a hotel room. Then I passed out for many hours. I was exhausted and finally had my first good sleep in days. I couldn't remember the last time I had slept for more than a few hours without interruption. Being on call for days and working at busy clinics had pushed me a little too far. The break was well earned—and the return trip with my family was refreshing and thankfully uneventful, which made me very happy.

My next adventure was a little scary for me as well as the other nurses. On a late afternoon, we received a visit by an expecting mum. This pregnant lady came in and she was in active labour. The delivery was imminent and was happening in the next few seconds. As the woman was placed on to a stretcher, the head was already coming out. We did our best to slow it down and control the delivery but that was not happening as it was too late. We needed her to come in about ten minutes sooner. We quickly suctioned a now crying baby that in one big push was out. After we made sure the baby was cleaned up and okay, we went to make sure mum was okay. That was when we realized we had a mess. My days in the OR were going to be my saving grace. With a rapid delivery, damage and tearing can happen all too easily. I had never seen it this bad before, so I was in a bit of shock, too. All I knew was that this was not good.

I started assessing the problem and I could see that the delivery was so forceful that the woman had received a very bad tear, which I classed as almost fourth degree, meaning she needed surgical intervention. After placing a call, the situation became even more serious. No planes could fly today and until the weather cleared there were none coming. Also, the ferry was out due to breakup so my plans for her to get to a surgeon were not happening. Plan A was out of the picture. Plan B was to do my best and start to put this mess back together again. It took me around two hours to clean, freeze and repair the tears and make the bleeding stop. After suturing and putting her back together as well as I could, I was so happy to see that the bleeding was controlled, the tissues all approximated and the damage was looking to be repaired. I had sutured multiple times in the past but this was by far my most complex case. Thank God for Dr. Ganguly explaining it to me and showing me the procedure back in the OR in Wetaskiwin. I may have never been able to attain my master's in nursing, and I also hadn't made graduating with a degree in nursing my priority, but I had an edge over most nurses. I had experience. I followed her recovery and was amazed at her quick recovery. In no time, she was back to 110 percent. Her little one did very well, too, and they soon were sent home and had no complications. All in all, things turned out okay, but it always made us all nervous when the unexpected happened.

In the north, we would run into the best people in the world. One fine day I met Elna, who was one of the most amazing nurses ever, for she came to be our charge nurse for a few months. The station ran like clockwork with her as our leader. Plus, we had more fun than anyone would have thought possible. One day Elna was helping me clean the pharmacy and I was looking after my son, JD. There was no really good place to put him, but Elna and I had a good plan. In no time JD was playing in the sink, he stayed in there for as long as we cleaned and got the place in top shape. We just kept him entertained with things around the station. Elna was also a diploma nurse, but she had been to many northern communities and had in the past been the acting director for the whole region. After our time, together in Fort MacPherson we have remained friends and I have kept in touch with the lady who was a mentor to me in so many ways.

One night we had to deal with a nasty fight. The police brought us in some patients from a domestic assault. Only one was a bloody mess: a sharp knife had been used to try and kill him. He had many stab wounds and the extra bleeding was washing out the stab wounds all too well. One of our nurses was in her own little world. She was busy going around offering nourishments and herbal tea to the police and staff who were rather busy. I went to work stopping the bleeding, cleaning, freezing, probing and making sure we could suture the stab wounds. Sometimes stab wounds are not sutured, as the rate of infection can be increased if they are, but if you don't they sometimes are reluctant or won't stop bleeding, so it's generally a good idea sooner than later to stop the blood loss. In no time, I had them all sutured up nicely. The medevac plane was delayed a few hours and the patient needed to be flown out ASAP as his injures were serious enough that he needed surgical consultation with possible intervention if a pneumothorax evolved.

Anytime you have stab or puncture wounds to the chest or the abdomen, or anywhere close to the retroperitoneal space in the back or even anywhere in the neck, you never know what could go wrong. They were never just something you could suture up and ignore as you never truly knew the depth or pathway of the weapon. Later on, we heard that this patient never needed a chest tube—nor, thankfully, a blood transfusion. We had no blood products anyway. We could draw the labs but not process them as we sent them to Inuvik to be processed by the proper lab staff. In a few hours, we had the assailant off to jail, and fortunately the RCMP were all safe tonight and back home within a few hours of the ordeal. We also had the victim sent off to the regional hospital safe and sound. It was a long night but a good night and no lives were lost.

Later I heard the nice doctor cut out every one of my sutures just to re-suture the wounds, as she didn't really like nurses all that much as we were performing many skills that some felt should only be done by a doctor. Many of the others doctors we worked with respected us greatly and were amazing on the other end of the phone on our many consults. We could order our own laboratory investigations and we would do our own X-rays, process our own X-rays and do our own referrals with no questions. We also made sure the patients always had the proper referrals if they needed them. About once a month we had a doctor come to the community and see our more complex patients, as we really strived to make their health the best it could be. They mattered greatly to us all. We had an incredible workload and it was a very challenging career. Once in a while we would get a new nurse and sometimes they were good and other times they were very bad. The bad ones were a problem for everyone in the community.

One sad night I was working a shift in the middle of the night when the police brought in a woman who had been raped. It was very violent and she was in shock. I assessed her immediately and made sure she was okay, ensured she didn't have any severe bleeding, ensured there was no immediate problems with her airway, breathing, and circulation (ABCs), as I was the nurse on call. That weekend I only had one other nurse in the community with me and we needed each other. I offered the victim a female nurse to perform the specialized assault examination as I felt it would be appropriate and that is what she requested. I was honestly very happy as I didn't want to do the rape examination as it was very invasive and a not nice procedure at any time. It was used to obtain evidence so the attacker could be charged and later convicted. Unfortunately, the exam can be nearly as traumatic for some people as the assault. It was such an emotional and hard examination for everyone involved. It was one of the hardest things I would do as a male nurse for obvious reasons.

I called the other on-call nurse who was being paid to be on call just like me. She answered and then told me she was too tired and hung up on me. She was a brand-new nurse to the community and my only other option that night. I was so angry. The police were even madder. They took my key and went up to the apartments above the nursing station and knocked and knocked on her door. She refused to open the door for them, as well. I wanted them to kick in her door but that was not a good idea. I was at a loss for a solution. I needed another nurse and tonight I needed a female nurse for obvious reasons. The police were also upset beyond belief; not mad at me, but at the predicament we all were in. The female nurse option was the right thing as it was the right thing for the patient. We also need the evidence and the rape exam had to be done ASAP and could only be done with the victim's consent. It meant flying the police plane from Yellowknife and picking up the patient and transporting her to another centre with an officer, or flying in a female nurse or physician to do the examination tonight.

I called the on-call senior administrator in the nursing office out of Inuvik. It was the middle of the night but she answered right away and was not mad at me but couldn't believe the situation. I offered to get the police to be more physical and she said, "No, Dale. That can't happen." She made a phone call to the local ER to check on the current staff and had a solution right away. They ended up chartering a special plane and put a nurse on it right away. The nurse working that night was a very good nurse and had packed her bags and was coming to our rescue. Thankfully the rape exam was done as required by a very caring female staff member and the patient was treated as humanly as possible. Most of all, she could see that we cared about her. It was a tragic night for all the staff. I know all the RCMP were also married and they too felt the pain in the night and only with the long hand of justice were they able to catch and convict the guilty party.

In the morning, the on-call nurse came downstairs and happily told me that she had a good sleep. I could have punched her in the head for the grief she'd caused us and that was not like me at all. But I just turned and walked the other way. Our new nurse that had been chartered in by plane was promoted to acting charge nurse and that was fine with me as I was really tired and I needed some sleep. I loved working as the staff nurse, anyway, much more than I enjoyed doing administration. Paperwork and staying in the office was not me. I only performed that role when it was needed of me.

The new charge nurse met the uncooperative nurse in the hallway at the start of the day. She was fired on the spot. She came up to me, crying, and told me she was sorry but she needed to sleep. I had no sympathy for her. Her days as a northern nurse were over forever. I understand we all have our breaking points but sometimes you need to go the extra mile, not just for the patients but also for your co-workers. I would have loved to sleep, too, but we had eight more hours of clinic and sick people to care for and then it would be time to get some rest. After all, sleep is overrated. I know when I'm dead and, hopefully, have gone to heaven, I'll be able to sleep all I want without pagers, radios or the telephone waking me up. The unfortunate nurse was escorted with her belonging to a waiting plane and was gone from the community.

When you live and work in a small community, you become respected by those living in the community. You help each other in their roles and as a team you make the community function even better. The one crazy thing I can remember doing "just because we could" was being sprayed by the local RCMP inspector with pepper spray, or OC spray, on purpose. A few of us nurses volunteered to attend the in-service training as it was now going to be mandatory for the RCMP to carry pepper spray, commonly referred to as OC spray. This was a very interesting experience but not one I'd like to repeat in this lifetime. It was instant fire in your eyeballs; your senses were all on fire and your desire to fight was instantly replaced with to the desire to drink something or wash your head with 3000 gallons of water.

The funny thing was I'd meet the instructor trainer of this course later on in a situation that made me hate a particular type of swarming insect even more than pepper spray. That day, I would get to see the RCMP inspector for the great leader and great father he was. After all it was a small world and the being up north it was smaller still.

We were called to a fatality on the Dempster Highway. I volunteered to go with the RCMP as soon as the call came in and off we went. Knowing it was going to be a body removal was not very reassuring, but we went just the same. It was a quiet ride to the scene and we really didn't say much. On arrival, we found a very sad scene. A nice, hard-working man had been hauling water for the Eagle Plains site when his water truck lost its air breaks coming down a steep hill. The truck driver tried to negotiate the steep curve at the bottom but the truck rolled and landed on the cab. Sometimes people and patients have no chance and this was one when airbags, seat belts had no real benefitted other than to keep the body in the cab when it was crushed. It was not a survivable event.

We tried to get access to get him out, but with the mangled truck on top of his cab we would need cutting tools, which were on their way but hadn't arrived yet. The RCMP had arranged for the Jaws of Life to be brought to us after the initial call and they were coming in by charter plane as soon as possible. While on scene, we heard the plane and an RCMP member went to meet it at a nearby runway. Not long after, we would get bad news. The plane could not see the runway due to fog. It was not safe to try and land so they aborted the landing and went back home with the Jaws of Life still on board. So, we needed to come up with another plan. We tried to lift the truck manually with jacks, and that was useless. Then the little bugs from hell started attacking us in waves. I guess they thought a dead person was an easy meal. Despite them trying to kill us we carried on. Giving up wasn't ever an option. No one was leaving this unfortunate man for insect bait. Somehow, someway, we would get him out.

The inspector for the RCMP was patrolling the Dempster Highway with the RCMP camper that day, and he and his kids stopped to help at the accident site. The gentle way he spoke to his kids and the authoritative, experienced tone he took on when he talked to the RCMP staff impressed me greatly. What an amazing man, but for the life of me I can't remember his name. Sometimes people are placed in this world for a specific reason. I would think it was destiny that everyone who was at the accident site was there that day.

Some calls were made and we located a payloader that could be brought to the scene, and that was about the only other way to get him out. It would need to lift up the large truck and then we would manually pull the victim out through the front or side window. The other RCMP had arrived from Dawson City with a simple coffin in the back of the police truck. The northern RCMP had some responsibilities that were not easy. This was a call not to be soon forgotten, but there were many honourable aspects about it, just the same. The RCMP were so dedicated to getting this man out, even though this wasn't their regular job. Normally, it would be the firefighters doing this type of work but in the north your job description is very diverse. In the end, we got him out and he was treated respectfully and carefully placed in the waiting temporary coffin, then sent off so the proper arrangements could be made.

After that day, I would have an increased respect for the work of the police and for their dedication to making this world a better place. I also felt a stronger bond with them and would always go out of my way to help them any chance I got. After that day, if I was in a drive-through and a police officer, RCMP or sheriff was behind me or in front of me, they got a free coffee or a meal. It was the least I could do for what they do for us every day. Somehow the police officer's role was much more diverse then most people would ever be able to comprehend.

The year I spent working as a community health nurse made me a much wiser person in many personal and professional pathways. From the visits with the patients to travelling the famous road from Dawson City to the top of the world I experienced so many unique events and experienced a much deeper respect for other cultures. A song that will always bring me back to those times is "Neil Colins" by a band called The Gumboots. The first time I heard it, I was at the Yellowknife airport on my way to Fort Good Hope in for a two-month position as a Charge Nurse at the local nursing station there. The lyrics of the song, which was about the Gwich'in people, rang so true to me.

The song was so true as they were such happy and caring people. The song almost made me cry for joy because Neil Colins story was almost not such a happy one if it was not for my timely interventions. In later years, whenever I would hear this song, I'd smile wide with my tonsils visible, thinking of the real Neil Colins and the memory I had of meeting him personally. I actually got to know him well and was partially credited for helping to save his life. Neil was as an elder from the Tetlit Gwich'in community, known as "The Mouth of the Peel" for his stories and dedicated work as an active radio host with CBQM radio in Fort McPherson. One day he was not feeling well and a home visit was requested. Another nurse had seen him and told him and the family that he was fine. The family called Mary, the CHR, and she asked me to come with her to Neil's house. When I walked into his home and took one look at him, I knew he was in trouble. You can judge trouble form a distance if you are always expecting it to be near.

Earlier that day the other nurse that had much more formal schooling than I did had performed a home visit and had declared him as ok. But I had the edge that no amount of education could reproduce. I'd seen thousands of sick and injured people throughout my relatively short career. I had learned to detect sickness and the look of death just coming from the doorway and looking in. It is something that can't be taught; experience teaches you to use your inner senses and apply common sense to the problems at hand. Also, you need to care about people and learn to feel their pain and see the unwritten or unstated signs of distress. That day, I knew right away we were in trouble. Neil was in trouble and time was already against us.

Before me, was a very nice, highly respected, Gwich'in elder. Neil was well known for hundreds of miles around as a happy and energetic person. This day I could see he wasn't the same. He had lost his shine. He was in severe pain but he would not complain. After I did a quick assessment, I said, "We're taking him to the nursing station." I was thinking it was likely an abdomen complication right from the start. To me, it appeared that was likely fighting a serious condition known as Systemic Inflammatory Response Syndrome or "SIRS." It was not sepsis, which is much worse, but most likely heading that way fast. If Neil crossed over toward the sepsis part of the illness, then he could easily die from irreversible shock.

I found from my head-to-toe exam that I was right. I had some working differential diagnosis and would not be 100 percent sure as we had no lab, no computer tomography (CT) scanners, no ultrasound (U/S), it was just experience and gut intuition making the diagnosis as accurate as possible. Just as I was getting ready to refer him to be flown out, the nurse who had seen him already came over to me and asked what I was doing and asked why I was sending him out. She then informed me she had her master's in nursing and that she was wiser than I was. I said that maybe she had more education but I had the experience, and I was going to ensure this man didn't die a slow, painful death. I was the charge nurse and I would look after it. If I turned out to be wrong, someone could reprimand me then. She went away mad. I helped to get Neil stable with IV fluid's and infused lifesaving antibiotics to bring on board to fight the suspected lethal infection coming, as well as administered Tylenol for pain and fever, and in no time, he was off in a medevac plane. If I was wrong, I was wrong, but if I was right and he was in trouble, he was on his way to safety. It would not be the first time a staff member was blind to the signs of trouble, and I would take the hit for that, too, but I would not let anyone die if it was an option.

In Inuvik, Neil was seen and assessed quickly and, sadly, I was right. By then he was in trouble and time was not in his favour.

So, he was packaged a second time and sent off to see the surgeon in Yellowknife. Thank God, he made it, and after several months of fighting for his life and slowly getting better, he was cleared to come back to his community. I was so proud the day he came to say thank you to me for saving his life. Then I knew I had made the right decision, despite my limited academic background. I would never be pushed aside and made to feel bad about being a nobody ever again.

I really worked hard to obtain my nurse practitioner (NP) title, but my provincial nursing body, CARNA, was never on my side. Fate was always against me getting ahead for some strange reason. I was prevented from getting the nurse practitioner title I should have had because I didn't have my masters. I tried to fight the system, but our nursing body took my money and stomped on my dreams and that was that. Looking back, they had set me up to fail by changing and making up rules up as they went. I'm sure a fellow nursing colleague who became a NP had thrown me under the bus, but it wasn't fatal. Just hurtful and sad to know what power does to people. It makes me happy to know I was not raised that way. After all, I was a nobody to them and they had the upper hand and the power to do what they wanted without appeal or reproach. Life has a specific purpose for each of us and we may never know where it will take us; we just need to ride along as far as the road takes us and get off at the right spot. The line from Joe in the movie Unconditional keeps coming back to me. "Life isn't a dead end if it takes you somewhere you needed to go."

Still, to this day, it hurts me to know how I was treated. But how they worked me over was much harder to swallow. In the end, though, I saved lives, and they made themselves feel better. I still win hands down. Despite the lack of the title and status, I can sleep better at night knowing my patients lived and the person who read my case studies likely never had half my experience. Just maybe they should have talked to me or walked a mile in my shoes! Funny thing was that the nurse who would have let Neil die is now a doctor, and I'm still a simple caretaker & lifesaver of thousands. Being a caretaker and lifesaver is my way of life, so that is just fine with me.

My leaving the North was not what I expected. On that day, as we were packing up, multiple community members arrived outside the nursing station and cried as they hugged me and said goodbye. I was so honoured to be so accepted and liked by a community that had taken me at face value and given me a chance. Once I proved myself and once they knew I cared about them, they were my friends for life. I had touched so many hearts, and they had made me a stronger and better person. On our drive home after Eagle Plains on our way down the Dempster Highway, we came across a giant moose. Just to see that beautiful animal close-up made my trip a paid-in-full adventure of a lifetime.

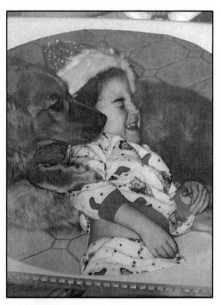

*"The Right People Make It Better"*

*Chapter 11: Challenging the Alberta System*

# "Fighting the System"

I always wanted to work EMS after nursing school and I had to find a way to do both as the pre-hospital care industry was in my heart for life. I thought there must be an easier way into the Alberta EMS System, as I didn't want to retake all the courses and start all over again. I just wanted to work extra, as having two or three jobs was what I did for fun. Working with the Wetaskiwin ER, and in the ambulance, we were lucky as we could use all of our skills and knowledge with no questions asked. When we worked as a registered nurses (RNs), we followed our nursing scope of practice, which basically meant we were supposed to do anything we could to get a patient from Point A to Point B alive.

We had licensed practical nurses (LPNs) and nursing aides (NAs) hired to drive one of the three units that were staffed by the hospital staff. Some of them were trained and had taken the Emergency Medical Technician (EMT) training and other were trained in first aid and CPR and held the appropriate driver's licence. For the most part, they were all very good at saving lives and had lots of practice making things right. Wetaskiwin had a way of making you gain experience in no time. You learned the hard way so many times, and you never forgot the lessons of life and death. We had many daily emergency calls and ALS transfers daily to all over the place. I just had to make the transfer some way from my minimal Saskatchewan training to graduating into my new system.

If I wanted to work in the local EMS, I need to be registered in Alberta and that wasn't as easy as you might think. In 1991, we had an ALS service taking over our local service and they would utilize me, but first I would need to jump through some hoops. I had to pass the provincial examination as an EMT and become registered to work. They let me start working as a registered nurse and gave me a chunk of time to get through the challenge and become registered. When the service started, I could work as an ALS attendant but I couldn't call myself a paramedic. That was okay with me, as I didn't care about the title; the chance to save lives and help others was my primary goal. My biggest thanks goes out to Carl Ringness and Bill Coghil for helping me through the red tape and hiring me into my first ALS position. They made it possible, and from then on forward I was one more step closer to my dreams.

My first hurdle was getting registered with the Alberta Paramedic Profession Association (APPA) to write the provincial examination. I had no idea it was so different from the Saskatchewan system. After that, I had to write the paramedic assessment examination to see where I stood in paramedic knowledge. I was lucky enough to pass it and the next hurdle was a bit harder. I had to go and perform a medical and trauma scenario—and I had no idea how to study for this or what to expect. So, I made the application and I showed up one fine Saturday, thinking I would have no trouble with this as I was already widely experienced, but sadly I was in for a shock. I failed the trauma scenario because I didn't know or wasn't prepared to recite the Basic Trauma Life Support (BTLS) parrot phrases while doing the head-to-toe examination. I had to say them in the right order or I would not get the points, and without the minimum points I would fail. Regardless of how good your patient care was, you had to follow the rules to pass a scenario and your real-world experience didn't hold any weight at all. I had to find a way to beat the game and I had less than twenty-four hours to figure out what I had to do to pass the scenario or redo the test next time around.

When they told me, I had to say the DCAP-BLS acronym, which stood for "Deformity, Contusions, Abrasions or Punctures" and then I had to feel or look for burns, lacerations or swelling, I must have looked dumb. I had never heard of this before that day. We never had BTLS courses in Saskatchewan prior to me moving to Alberta. Plan B was to find a book and figure it out fast. I had to get it done before tomorrow. They were giving me one chance for a redo trauma scenario. I wasn't going to quit my dream that day, so somehow, someway, I had to find a way to beat the system.

As soon as I got back to Wetaskiwin, I went to the local hospital library and searched for the BTLS textbook. In no time, I had found it. Thankfully, it was only ninety-three pages long. Yes, we had a chance and tomorrow I would get one more chance to make it. That night, I read the book cover to cover and before the next day I had the BTLS phrases memorized. I had to get someone to cover my shift until I was done with the exam and as soon as I got through it I would go back to my real job. That day was one I will never forget. My partner was the most amazing EMT in the world. He was the strongest and biggest EMT I'd ever seen. Darren was the gentle giant and always gave his patients the best care possible. I had no idea then that one day in the future he would be lost in a training accident after he became a Calgary Police officer on a swat training exercise.

I got the scenarios done and came right home and went straight back to my shift. Darren was my partner and, after a stressful testing day, I was lucky to have him at my side. Every time we sat down that day to eat, the tones would go off. We would go to the next emergency call, pick up and transport the patient to hospital and then we would be ready to do it all over again. The third time the tones went off that day, we knew it was going to be the bad call that we all wanted but dreaded at the same time. It would be the call to prove ourselves. We were dispatched to a collision between a freight train and a minivan. It would stretch us all to the limits of our caring ability and prove why team members need to work as one to get through calls and save as many lives as possible. We couldn't save everyone that day, but we gave one hundred and ten percent effort to them all with the time we had and sometimes time is all we can give. That evening we lost three people who were at the wrong place at the wrong time. A few seconds was all they would have needed for the speeding train to miss them, but it hit the car right in the middle of the driver's door. Immediate death was likely a gift for mother that day for her injuries would all be incapable of living.

The accident was a level crossing about seven miles north of town. Off we went with the siren screaming and the lights making everyone see we were coming past. We had reached our maximum speed in no time. The lines in the road looked like dots. I remember looking back behind me and we had three RCMP cars rapidly gaining on us. I was already going one hundred miles an hour (160 km), passing and meeting vehicles, and they passed me as if I wasn't even moving. It was breathtaking. On arrival, we found complete chaos and a big mess. We were told the train was going so fast it had hit the minivan and pushed it down the tracks over a half a mile, or about one kilometer. The train had hit the van at a level crossing and simply pushed it down the tracks without it exploding or coming apart. The minivan was wrapped around the front engine and was a mangled mess. I thought to myself that it would be a miracle if anyone survived this horrific accident, as I grabbed our trauma kits and took off at a dead run for the minivan.

We had multiple police helping us and the fire crews were coming. You could hear the sirens of many emergency vehicles in the distance. The cavalry was on its way. The biggest problem was we only had one other EMS unit coming for backup. The other unit was on another call and was trying to get back to help us in the next few minutes. I found an unconscious child in the front seat, pinned under his dead mum. The driver's side of the van and been pushed in so far it had molded the front bucket seats together. The mother had taken the brunt of the force on her driver's door and nothing could have saved her that fateful day. Her son had his leg trapped between the van's bucket seats and we could not release it. Thankfully, he was unconscious. To wake up and see your mum dead on top of you would have been horrific. I know the mother gave her life for him as she took the brunt of the force of the lateral impact. Thankfully, her son had a chance to live because of her last gift of life.

In the backseat of the minivan we had two other patients. A young boy on the passenger side and a girl on the driver's side just behind her mother. The boy was hit so hard his cranium was split and shifted. It was a very serious head injury but he was alive, his breathing was adequate and he had a strong bounding pulse. Next to him was his sister, Krista, who I looked after the most. Krista must have turned her head and looked at the train as it hit them. She was completely broken and her face and head were a total mess. She was moaning slightly. Constable Ben Draper of the RCMP, who was a good friend of mine, was my helper. We slid Krista out of the van and took her immediately to the unit. One of the EMTs stayed with her and I went back to grab the boy from the front seat. Another crew member had grabbed the boy from the backseat already. I had to get the boy out from under his mum and get going to the local ER or his sister would die waiting for help. We had no more people to help. I had to get him out now. Ben and I did everything we could to release his trapped leg. The fire department was just setting up but I didn't have time to wait for the Jaws of Life to do their magic.

I started pulling as hard as I could on his trapped leg. Ben was helping and it would not move. I then realized the weight of his mother wasn't helping us get him out. Mum had saved him from the impact, but now we had to get her off him. I grabbed her and started pushing her head, neck and back to move her off her son. I've never seen the bucket seats so molded together in the front before and creating such an unforgiving vise effect. Slowly, she shifted, and I told Ben, "You pull that leg out and if we break it then we break it. We've got to leave now." We had no more time. Krista needed me and we could not wait for the Jaws or the local fire department to free the leg. It was life over limb time. Ben pulled and I pushed and all a sudden the leg released itself. We rapidly slid him out onto a spine bard and he went right to our unit and was placed beside Krista who was waiting for my interventions if at all possible. I had my work set out and no time to make decisions. I just had to do what I could do in a timely fashion. This one call was what made us earn the right to call ourselves a paramedic.

I could stay on scene and try to intubate her or we could make a mad dash for the local ER. I had attended a very good trauma course in the USA in 1986 and I was very aware that time was already against us all. One rule that they taught us was if you're less than seven minutes from a hospital with a bad trauma, the hospital is your friend. You loaded the patient and got there as fast as possible. It cut down your golden hour. Today it could and would be the right answer in my mind that was traveling at the speed of light.

At the end of the day in any serious patient you just needed to have an adequate airway, a palpable pulse and you could keep your patient alive for long enough to get to more help. Krista needed the airway and I needed expert help to get it right the first time. I thought about it quickly. I grabbed the mic and called the local ER. I told them we were in-bound with two critical pediatric patients and needed anesthesia waiting for us on arrival. We would be there in less than seven minutes. We had two unconscious kids in our unit, one with a bad airway, and I had no time to try to be a hero and intubate myself.

We didn't have the right medications and expert help was mere minutes away. I wasn't going to take a chance and make the wrong decision, as I had two lives in the balance. We were off like a bullet. The siren screamed and split the traffic in two and we were making the transfer to the closest ER at the speed of our red and blue lights, or it sure seemed that way that fateful night. We needed one thing for sure before we go there and I was going to get it. An intravenous for medications was mandatory. I could not miss this one. Krista needed an advanced airway and her life depended on it.

After we pulled away, I grabbed an angiocath and I found a vein that was going to be my target. I applied the tourniquet and said a prayer out loud, "God help me." I slipped the IV into Krista's vein in a few seconds. Normally I put in the angiocaths slowly, but today I just drove it into her vein right to the hub of the needle. This was not my normal way, but it was not a normal situation. I knew we could then get an advanced airway. With the right people, the right drugs and the right atmosphere, we were set up to win. All things were possible with lifesaving IV access.

Intubation is experience and skill combined. I made one attempt to intubate her but she was biting enough that I couldn't get the laryngoscope in far enough to get the cords into view as we were driving to the hospital. Her upper and lower jaw and face were broken badly and she was biting down on me enough that it would not be easy even for an expert. Looking down at her split face and knowing she was someone's shining little lady broke my heart. Thankfully, when we rolled into the ER they were ready. Dr. Argals, our local anesthesiologist, was waiting for us. It would turn out to be his finest hour.

As soon as we rolled in the door, the right medications were called for and within a few minutes we had a better and secure airway. I will never forget that it was a simple medication recipe. Just one drug, as it was quick and available. The anesthesiologist used Demerol in 10 mg increments and he kept repeating it until she was relaxed, and in no time, you could see her fight was gone and then she settled enough that we could ventilate her properly and the endotracheal tube was slid right in on the first attempt. After just a few ventilations, her chest was rising correctly and her oxygen saturations were climbing. It was so amazing to see a really bad airway go to one with a small magic tube misting with every exhalation. "Krista, you have a chance," I whispered. Little did I know it wasn't going to be for long. Her destiny was already decided.

The whole time I was helping to intubate, I was not aware I was stepping on a nurse's foot. I was trying to lift Krista's mangled jaw in just the right direction and we were suctioning out a path to place the little uncuffed endotracheal tube, so I was oblivious to everything else. Barb never said anything until the endotracheal tube went past the vocal cords and then she said ever-so-nicely, "Get off my foot." Many years later, Barb took her own life and I know it was most likely related to the repeated evil she saw at work for too many years. Barb was also a mother of two kids and I'm sure seeing situations like this wasn't easy on her. No one is immune to the broken faces and the repeated pain inflicted on others day after day.

I was so thankful I had made the right decision and come to the closest hospital and that help was ready and waiting. Now we had three kids that needed a pediatric trauma centre and STARS was not an option. They were using a smaller helicopter, a single-pilot BO-105, and it flew out of the Edmonton Municipal Airport. It was only able to fly during daytime hours and it was already past dusk. As I thought about it, I realized that the sunset had likely caused this accident. The sun would have been right in the mother's eyes and she probably hadn't seen the train until it was too late. Normally, we think of the sun as giving life, but a few times in my life I would see it also gave death.

After the kids were stabilized we needed to get them to the best trauma centre possible. They all needed much more critical care and help than any of us could provide and time wasn't on our side. We elected to load all three kids in our unit and take off for the trauma centre. We would actually pass the train and minivan crash site on the way.

Bill was our driver and he was the best of the best. We had two very good EMTs on board and me as the paramedic in the back with Bill guiding our unit past many potential disasters down the highway and through the city traffic. En route, we met another unit and used their cardiac monitor to help us monitor the three critical kids on the drive over. It was not a long trip but the forty-five minutes it took seemed like a lifetime to me.

Looking back, it was one of the busiest transfers of my career. I will never know how, but we got all three kids to the Pediatric Trauma Centre at the University of Alberta alive. The problem was we had three broken kids and only two spots in the unit. Darren, using his strength and wisdom, used his knees to hold the end of the middle spine board up for the whole trip. The top half was wedged between the stretchers. It wasn't legal, but we did it anyway. In times of a multiple casualty incident (MCI) or a disaster, the rules were different. I was thinking that tonight was a mini disaster, so we didn't have to follow the rules. "Better to seek forgiveness then seek permission" was an unwritten rule that I had used over and over again and which had helped make a difference in many outcomes.

On arrival, the University of Alberta Hospital / Stollery staff swarmed us in the ambulance bay. They rapidly took over our critical patients and our job was done. They took Krista away from us and I thought maybe we had a performed a little miracle. The kids were all alive and we had made the trip in record time. We had been pushed to our limits and triumphed over one of our worst days. Our job was done but our brains and our thoughts were far from slowing down. I had so many what-ifs swirling around in my head that night. I still had five patient care reports (PCRs) to write and I had not done one yet. It was a going to be a long night.

I had slept minimally the night before and had been up since 5:00 a.m. and I still had another four or five hours left before I could sleep as I was on shift until 7:00 a.m. I knew I would make it, but I just didn't know how. The song "Only God knows Why" by Kid Rock still makes me think back to this call. It is so emotional when you see this type of tragedy over and over. All we can do is do our best and help the ones we can, and let the others go.

Tonight, we had done the unthinkable and everyone from Ben on scene to Barb the ER RN to Dr. Argals as everyone else involved made a difference to try to save three separate lives. Even with our personal loses adding up over the years we just kept fighting the next loss, and we took everyone just as hard as the one before. That's what makes a difference: it was the team's loss and not any one person's. We all did our best and as a team we all felt the loss.

Very sadly, an hour after we left the Stollery and had started back home to clean up our mess, Krista passed away, and by the next morning they had also lost her little brother. The only one to make it was her brother who had been sitting in the front seat after his mum gave her life for him. I know in my heart the mother gave her life for that child so he could live. I heard later that the poor dad was called from a curling bonspiel to the hospital only to learn the worst news imaginable. I'm sure he's still hurting today and will never be the same without his kids and his wife. Today he was granted the life of one child and even with the severe loss it would be still a small miracle.

I guess if nothing else, we gave him a little more time with his broken family to say goodbye. We had given him more time to get to their side to say what needed to be said. We had pushed the limits and bought them just a little more time and that was all we could have done in the face of such overwhelming odds.

A short time later, we received a letter addressed to our local ambulance service. It was a commendation letter for the excellent care we had provided to the kids that tragic Sunday evening. The staff had reported us to the hospital management team. The staff in the ER along with the doctors, the RTs and the nurses had seen our hearts ripped to shreds as we were doing our best despite the odds. They could see and feel how hard we had worked to try to save those children. We pulled out every possible procedure from our wisdom to help save lives even if it was only for a short time it was still something.

I realized after that day that I wasn't good enough to pass an Alberta Prehospital Providers Association (APPA) test as an Emergency Medical Technician, as I was unable to recite the parrot phrases, but I got a letter of commendation for helping to save real lives. I helped extricate, transport, and stabilize those children in spite of being told that I wasn't good enough. We had achieved our goal of keeping those broken and critically injured children alive long enough to get to a trauma centre. That's the day I realized that sometimes APPA testing and the current structure was just part of this game of life. I passed the real test, but the simulated ones at AAPA had not gone so well. You just have to know that all games have rules and, just like in baseball, you have to follow the rules after you hit the ball in fair territory. You actually need to touch the bases on a home run or you're out, regardless of how far you hit the ball or how fast you can run.

I never forgot how hard everyone had worked that day to make a difference in the outcome that day. Ben, my RCMP friend, was at my side the whole time and would have done anything to help get those kids safely to our unit. The other staff on the call were all equally amazing. The hospital staff at WGH and the Stollery had done an excellent job as well. We faced that situation as a team. That one call will always be the one call that made me know we must work as a team to help save lives. Team work is essential for our survival as well.

Several years later I would be tested again. I challenged the APPA paramedic status next, and I did okay on the written examination but again I had to do scenarios. Scenarios were going to be the death of me. I had the misfortune of getting sick shortly before. I needed to see a doctor as I was not feeling well and ended up having to get my appendix out five days before the scenario testing. It turned out that my abdominal pain was due to an acute appendix attack.

This was not good news. I could not be having an appendix attack as I was getting ready for the APPA scenarios and I knew from my last experience that they would be trying to fail me from the start. This wasn't helping my confidence level at all. I was admitted to the hospital and sent for emergency surgery. Tina Pederson, who was my partner on many calls and also my friend, looked after me for the transfer, which made me feel a little better knowing that I meant so much to her. I just knew when she held my hand and looked into my eyes that I was someone special to her. We both shed a few tears when she dropped me off at the urban hospital to go directly to the next available operating room (OR). It was time for me to be a patient and not the health care worker.

The surgery went well despite the terrible care I received on the ward after the surgery. I had one visit by a nurse on the day shift and then a doctor came and told me I could go home. I asked him if they would mind covering my open abdomen or put a dressing over it. They Steri-Stripped it shut and by 4:00 p.m. I was picked up and taken home. No pain medications and no antibiotics for an infected appendix I thought was almost as bad as you could get. My family took me back to Wetaskiwin, and my friend Dr. Idicula fixed me up with the right medications and home I went. I was sick and not well for several more days.

Looking back to my first surgical misadventure, the recovery room staff at the Grey Nuns was so amazing and so caring. I can remember them worrying as my blood pressure was so low, but I didn't care as I knew I was going to live despite being so sick. That week after my surgery I was not a very sociable or caring person as I felt so sick. I was so sick I couldn't drive myself to my provincial Alberta College of Paramedics (ACP) paramedic scenario exams in Calgary about 5 days later. So, I made a call and my good friend Eileen Chambers agreed to take me to the examinations. I was stoned on Darvon and did not do well enough to pass my medical call. They failed me, but I wasn't about to quit. Quitting was not an option. I had Jamie, Burt and many other guardian angels there to pick me up. I was their avenging angel. I fought evil at all levels. Someone had to help me up and I don't think I would have had the power on my own. Everyone has a breaking point. I needed my friends to help me get going and over time I realized it was not my fault I failed and I knew I would just redo the practical exam and next time I would win at any cost.

Later, I would see first-hand the broken system with Alberta College of Paramedics (ACP) stuck in the Health Disciplines Act (HDA). We should have been in the Health Professions Act (HPA) many years ago. We would be helpless to change it for the next fifteen years. We had good students fail and poor students make it through. We had many debates with the system and slowly we made it better but never fixed the original system. We just learned how to fight the system most times, and that was all we could do for many of our students.

Even today, the system isn't right and I had to give up trying to change it from the outside as it seemed like I was wasting my time and effort. I needed to just worry about the things I could change or fix and ignore the stuff that I couldn't. If you can't fix it or change it, sometimes the only way you can sleep at night is to walk away from it. I walked away on my terms.

Sadly, over the years we keep eating our own to prove something to others. It seems as if we treat new people in EMS like they are nothing until they can prove themselves. It should be that we all support one another and operate as a team. Sadly, that isn't the way it is yet in EMS, especially in our current ambulance model. Fire, as well as police welcome new people more openly. They have a mentorship model that works. We need to change the system so that the initial probationary period is set up more like a mentorship. We need to support our new members and ensure they have a role model to lead them to be successful.

Can you imagine if everyone on the team actually wanted you to succeed? Everyone would be better for the support in the end. More experienced professionals would learn the newest practices and wisdom from their students, so it would be a win-win. Team building and morale building is never a waste of time or effort at any level.

I have not totally given up but I can say I'm frustrated with a system that needs to build from within. But as soon as I get my second wind I will change the system. I know this as I've already made a big dent in EMS in my short lifespan. One step at a time we will make the system better. Or, I might just die trying and that's okay, too. I'd rather die fighting the good fight then watch the world go to pot. Maybe by making my books in the future we can help bring our EMS world to new increased heights.

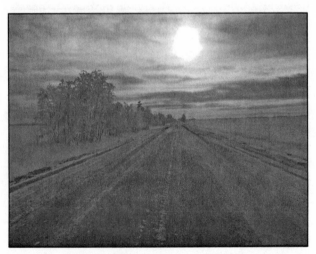

*"Always Look for the Best in the Worst"*

# "Team Effort"

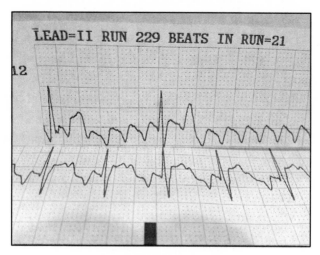

*"Teaching the Right Stuff"*

I have spent over twenty years teaching all the different EMS programs in Alberta. The personal challenges are very rewarding with being an instructor. The more effort you put into the students, the more they would benefit. I'm sure some of my grey hair came from wondering if we taught the students enough. They needed to know everything there was to know in order to make the right decisions on every call and in every situation. I was lucky, as I was just one of the teachers that made some of the best professionals in the Emergency Medical Services.

At other schools, I had seen some instructors who called themselves teachers but who were just there to pad their own resumes. The good ones were there to teach and share not only their knowledge but their wisdom. I've met many instructors who put their heart and soul into every class they teach and they are the ones the student won't ever forget. We were all just the right stuff as teachers.

At Augustana University College and then Lakeland College we had the right, dedicated instructors to help our students succeed in the EMS world. We all had our strengths and weaknesses, but as a team, we worked better then you could imagine. I sincerely believe we were meant to be together at that specific time and place. When you have a winning team behind you, it's hard to lose. If I could go back and change anything it would be to fight even harder to keep our team together even longer. When you personally know the best and work with the best, your results will reflect that as well. I've never know any other EMS school to have such a good team in my entire EMS career.

For years, Debbie Smeaton was responsible for keeping us all on the straight and narrow educational road of life. We had many others who made up the winning team including Tim Essington, Len Stelmaschuk, Heather Verbaas, Cheryl Cameron, Tanya Blades, Wes Baerg, Dan Schmick and Kevin Sitter. I started with the Augustana University College EMS teaching team in 1999 and ended with the Lakeland team in 2013 when the campus was closed in Camrose. We as a team embarked on a long successful career to make the best Emergency Medical Responders (EMRs), Emergency Medical Technicians (EMTs) and finally Emergency Medical Technologist – Paramedics in the province and we did it. Our legacy of success will never be forgotten by the few that made it all possible.

Most of our success was demonstrated in the results of our students in the industry. After they graduated, many would spread their wings and seek higher levels of education. Many now have degrees and some have achieved their master's. For many that would not have been possible before graduating from the paramedic program. Our success stories exceeded our own expectations by far.

Right from the early days, Tim Essington, who was the head instructor of the first Distance EMS Paramedic Program at Alberta Vocational College (AVC-Lac La Biche) and then with Augustana University College, knew we needed a distance education program that would ensure rural EMS members had the same high-quality training as EMS members in urban centres. Tim had the vision and could see the need for Advanced Life Support education in rural areas just as much as it was needed in the cities. The in-house programs were not a possibility for many who could not afford to take two years off to go to Northern Alberta Institute of Technology (NAIT) or Southern Alberta Institute of Technology (SAIT). A Distance Paramedic Program was a dream come true for many students as well as for the instructors that believed in this methodology right from the start of the idea through to its inception.

This made it possible for rural students to get their education over the intranet along with scheduled on-site days and technical weeks at Camrose. On those teaching weeks, students would attend for approximately five days and go then go home. The students worked hard and many of them socialized hard, as well, during the intense week. It was not uncommon for me to meet several of them at the school or at Starbucks for some extra help. The topics we discussed ranged from cardiology to pharmacology. Several students told me later on that these extra sessions were what saved them.

I wanted to ensure they my students always had someone they could call on. "Leave no one behind" was my personal motto. All the students had my number and my email so they could get in touch with me 24/7. If I didn't know the answer to one of their questions, I would find someone who did. It was not uncommon for me to be the lone person corresponding with students through the intranet software at 3:00 a.m., trying to get a teaching point across. When I was sure the student had what her or she needed, I would go to sleep again. Many times, they were almost at the right answer but just needed a push to make the final leap. It was a bit like getting ready to parachute from a plane: you have the means to do it, but you need to pull the cord at the right time. You are responsible for ensuring you pull the right cord, but heaven forbid a problem arises, then you still have your emergency chute. One of us instructors would then rescue you.

We also dealt with student emergencies that were not your typical fare. Breakups and family emergencies were common, and those we dealt with as a team. In one case, a student came to us and we realized he needed to go to a treatment program right away. In our line of work, we see the worst of the worst. This student needed help, and we would have moved heaven and earth for him. We helped get him admitted right away and he got the help he needed. I know his success in our program was partly due to the fact we had his back when he needed us.

I know some of his pain was from taking EMS calls. In a typical day, we may go from trying to save someone who has third degree burns to ninety per cent of his body to attending to a call from a dad who has accidentally run over his two-year-old in the driveway. Those calls never leave you. They are yours to keep forever. Every time I came across this former student at work, I give him a hug and they also know that I'm proud of them for making this world a little bit of a better place.

If you decided to try to sail through school and not apply yourself and do the bare minimum to get by, you were off my list. There was always the odd student who would not work out well in this profession for a variety of reasons. The good ones who have carried on my legacy are mentioned in the back of my book in the "Dedication" section. They have made the required effort and deserve the right to hold the title they now hold.

When my students were successful, it was a fulfilling sensation. It was a privilege to know they were now part of my EMS family for life. The sweat and tears paid off for every student who applied him or herself. Over the years, I have made special friends who will always be on my contact list and with whom I'll always keep in touch. If they need help or I need help, we are just a call away from each other.

The hardest part about teaching is getting the message across at the right level for the students to understand. Every student has unique abilities and some have unique learning disabilities, as well. You need to be able to transmit the necessary knowledge in a form that they can properly digest in order to be able to apply it as needed. As EMS workers, sometimes we have time to react and sometimes we don't, so decisions must be fast, calculated and right most of the time.

We all have special students throughout our careers that we won't ever forget. I know Tim and many other instructors would agree that Rixford Smith was one student who deserved to be a paramedic, but getting him to that level was not easy. The road may have been longer for Rixford, but the end results were lifelong and are still seen in his excellent interactions with patients. Today Rixford is a practitioner who excels in patient care despite the ever-changing Alberta Health Services (AHS) and Alberta College of Paramedics (ACP) education requirements. I am always fearful that he will be slowly forced out for not meeting the current requirements of the system.

I was so fortunate to teach one student right from the time of her high school graduation through the Emergency Medical Responder (EMR) course then the Emergency Medical Technician – Ambulance (EMT-A) program, and finally the Emergency Medical Technician – Paramedic (EMT-P) program. Heather would be the youngest person to ever graduate as a paramedic in the province of Alberta. Many people never knew the battles she had faced as a student. Today she is one proud, successful woman. Heather was motivated and determined to be the best of the best. The first day I met her I saw something special in her, as it was clear she wanted to help people and was not in it for the glory or the money. It was almost as if she had made up her mind at a young age of where she was going in life and was determined that it would happen no matter what obstacles she encountered. For me she was and will always be an angel. God only makes a few people of her calibre, and they are out in this world, putting up a good fight.

In EMS, there are many rites of passage that are earned the hard way and not always the right way. If you earn your strips or badges along the road of life you own those accomplishments, as well. We would see many students who would need to fight the still- male-dominated system. There are still services out there today where female members are not treated equally, but things are a lot better than they were in the past. I had to face similar discrimination as a male nurse.

Many people in our industry are intimidated by people they know are going to be successful. I will never know why some people think it's their right to preside as the judge and jury over someone else's education. I have seen many students discriminated against and treated poorly by instructors who were completely in the wrong. Apparently, they never got the memo that they were supposed to be mentors to their students, not act as roadblocks to their success.

Then along came Rixford, who is one of my students that I have always kept in touch with from the first time we met on the highway after he placed a call for an Advanced Life Support (ALS) backup.

Rixford is a believer and always will be as that is the type of a person he was raised to be. Rixford was born into a wonderful Christian family with very strong moral and ethical beliefs that exceeded those of many others. Rixford lived and breathed his beliefs but never pushed them on anyone. He was simply a man on a mission.

When I first met Rixford, he was working with a local Basic Life Support (BLS) ambulance service. I could see his dedication and his desire for higher learning. I would help him on his patient care reports after the calls and tried to keep him on the road to success. I never knew back then that his life goal was actually to launch a missile into space, but regardless, he was a unique and brilliant young man. The more you learn about people, the more you realize why they were put on this earth and that we all have a unique purpose in life.

Rixford had personally known discrimination from a young age. Rixford had very severe dyslexia to the point that many of his teachers thought he was stupid. Dyslexia would always be a hurdle for Rixford, even if he was gifted in many other aspects of his life. Rixford would likely not get through any other EMS paramedic program as most instructors would consider him unteachable.

We had several students in every class who had learning disabilities. As a school, we challenged the provincial exam to be changed for this reason; it wasn't fair for those with learning disabilities. A learning disability shouldn't prevent you from being successful in life. As people, we all have our strengths and weaknesses. Luckily, we got the exam changed. As with everything, the EMS world is a changing system and most times the system is changed for the better.

The accommodations were a lifesaver for the students who deserved them. For example, one student whom I had been helping would be overcome with exam anxiety. To this day, Kim will always be my hero for never quitting. Every time she was knocked down, she'd get back up fighting. That's what makes a winner. Winners are fighters.

The people against changing the old system were in the minority. The schools that had Rixford kicked out due to his learning disability should be ashamed to be in this industry.

Thank God, Rixford found some educators who had a vision, and with them on his side, there was no stopping him.

Rixford and I had a close bond right off the top for a few reasons right. Rixford's Achilles heel was basically the same as mine: he would do fine on the practical part of the paramedic exam but the scenario-based testing was not as easy for him. When it came to the scenario testing, he had trouble as he was treating a real patient in his head and the testing was a scenario and they are so different and not very practical. That was when I stepped up to rescue him. I worked with him to get him to think of how to play the scenario game and ensure he could make the best choice in a simulated event.

Rixford had achieved a passing mark on the written portion of the provincial exam; they had provided him with the appropriate accommodations. All he needed was to succeed at the scenario game. Our examiners at the time were always happy to let people miss something they considered a serious error and then they could fail them. It drove me mad. Over the years, we had many students who played the scenario right but still failed as they didn't follow the particular set of steps the examiners were looking for.

Rixford was just one more student who made it hard for me to look the other way when the system was unjust. The current testing system was flawed, as it was not the true picture of the ability of the student to be a professional. It never evaluated competence. It only showed that they could pass or fail a simulated scenario. I would later see many students' pass a scenario but be completely lost when it was time to apply their knowledge on a critical call.

The real world and the scenario world were never the same and will never be the same evaluation. We need to change our testing and evaluation system to demonstrate this in the future if we want to survive as a profession. The success of our EMS profession is directly related to our evolution as people in a unique trade and with a unique skill attainment. The ability to pass a scenario proves nothing about actual competence or skill integration in the real world. That was what made me upset: it was not a logical system and was not set up for transparency at all levels of testing, which was mandatory.

One day they started failing students for not using dopamine in a trauma scenario. In the pre-hospital world, you should never use dopamine as a first-line treatment; rather, you would always use IV fluid along with repeated boluses and then blood products, if available, first. After reviewing several of their scenarios, it was clear the scenarios were flawed on many levels.

I was the pharmacology instructor for our students before graduation, plus I worked as a critical care nurse and as a paramedic, so I had some expertise with medications. I had used dopamine on many cases. Plus, I was familiar with multiple other pressor agents that ACP was still not ready to use as they were slow about change. I had seen dopamine used wrongly in trauma cases in the past and it was always a bad outcome if patients were wrongly treated or under-treated while in a state of shock. I knew that one of the harmful side effects of dopamine was an increased tachycardia, as well as increased BP, which was not a good thing if the patient was still bleeding or had an unstable bleed.

When dopamine was used in a hypovolemic patient it would just drive up the heart rate and enhance bleeding. The faster the heart rate and the more forceful the contractility of the heart muscle, the faster the rate of blood loss in patients with uncontrolled bleeding.

Some of the scenarios these examinations contained were so unrealistic and the people making them up so unwise to the real world of critical care medicine. As instructors, we were teaching our students that sometimes we desired the patient to have permissive hypotension. This means we allow the BP to be lower than normal, especially in an uncontrolled bleeding condition. If we added dopamine it could increase the heart rate BP, which in turn could worsen any uncontrolled bleeding in the chest. As the pressure increases, patients bleed more and more in proportion to the increased pressure gradient. Many of these patients end up needing urgent surgical interventions.

One way I would get this point across to my students was by explaining it like this: Just think of the patient as having a little pinhole in their garden hose. As the pressure increases, the leak greatly increases. If you step on the hose just past the hole, the water sprays even harder as it takes the path of least resistance. This is similar to how bleeding works and is demonstrated in hemorrhagic shock. It all comes down to physics and flow. As in almost everything, common sense plays an important part of medicine. But we sometimes don't rely on common sense enough in emergency medicine.

We would try to teach our students some simple concepts such as the four components needed to consider in patients in hypovolemic shock. With shock, you will always see one of four problems in the patient. One of these is hypovolemia, which is purely a volume problem. Hypovolemic shock can cause many other complications in the body due to lack of perfusion, which also affects cellular respiration.

Then we often see a heart rate problem—mostly tachycardia, but younger patients can demonstrate a bradycardia rhythm or a lower heart rate than you would expect. In elderly or older patients on beta blockers, this side effect can be masked and you will see even worse hypotension with a normal heart rate. The next one we would consider is pooling of fluid in the extremities or the lack of a vascular tome that helps to maintain an adequate BP. The last and most important consideration would be the ability for the heart to be an effective pump.

A good teaching point I will never forget comes from the MASH treatment era. Military medicine has taught us some good and bad lessons. The best lesson I can think of is related to trauma care and the complications from our care or interventions. During the Vietnam War, there were many patients in very bad condition from bleeding and significant blood loss. Many patients' BP would drop down to around 40 systolic for long periods of time. In some cases, the patients had to wait one to two days before being medevacked or treated.

Although their BP stayed critically low, they didn't die right away under certain bleeding conditions. Everyone wondered why their BP went to 40/systolic and just hovered, but then someone figured it out: Bleeding is pressure or volume-related. If you have a low BP or a no blood-pressure situation, then you will have a minimal or no-bleeding situation. Low capillary pressure and bleeding stops and clotting or hemostasis can occur.

They noticed in these military shock patients that if you pushed the patients past their limits, they would bleed out or finally end up in cardiorespiratory arrest. The medics could provide some basic care to help treat the shock but over time the clotting and compensation mechanism would fail. Sick patients who went on to develop decompensated shock followed then by multiple organ dysfunction syndrome, known as MODS are the patients we will not be able to save despite our best interventions. If we just let them rest and be severely hypotensive, they still had a chance to survive. This was when they found the patients didn't bleed out when their BP got very low as they had no pressure to bleed. They noted that when BP was low, capillary pressure was also low and you need increased pressure to bleed so therefore low BP is sometimes helpful in trauma cases.

We know from modern medicine the higher the BP, this increased the bleeding is in many cases. There has been a shift in the last several years for us to utilize permissive hypotension on certain cases in International Trauma Life Support (ITLS) and Advanced Trauma Life Support (ATLS). This is the same logic that the Alberta

College of Paramedics ACP, or the provincial exam, was not so keen on.

As a teacher, I would see scenarios so far out of left field it was impossible to win. Some scenarios had no actual concrete rationale or reason to their logic. They were impractical and impossible scenarios that contraindicated the ATLS or critical care treatments of today. The province had taken the scenario world to an all-time low. I told my students who failed these scenarios to appeal, as they were not even a real option for a paramedic. We needed to treat a patient and not a scenario, and with that there should always be some flexibility.

One day, a group of us instructors were sitting in a staff meeting when we were interrupted for the best reason ever. The local EMS providers came in for Advanced Life Support (ALS) help. This happened when a Basic Life Support (BLS) unit was in trouble and they needed help right away. They had been called to a severe stabbing that was beyond their scope of expertise and we were just a call away.

Tim Essington and I were picked up and taken to a fully stocked ALS unit. We hit the lights and kicked the siren on and we were off as quick as possible, headed to the location of the stabbing. We knew the police were also backing us up, so it was all good. Before arrival we heard it was now a cardiac arrest.

If it was a cardiac arrest and related to a stabbing, it had to be one of the serious situations we all referred to as the Deadly Dozen. Our patient was most likely in hypovolemic shock, and a tension pneumothorax, hemopneumothorax or possibly cardiac tamponade was most likely the reason for the cardiac arrest, but we wouldn't know for certain until we arrived on scene. On a call like this, your mind is always searching for differential diagnosis and you want to make sure you can rule them out as quickly as possible.

It was not often that two instructors could show up and assume control and rock a call, but we would try our best. Tim was my friend, my coworker, my boss and also my partner for years back when we worked in Wetaskiwin together. We had done hundreds of EMS calls and transfers together. We worked very well as a team and we knew each other's strengths and weaknesses. Before arrival, we had a plan of attack. We always had a plan. Plan A was for Tim to intubate while I got the IVs in and running right away, as that was my specialty. If Tim had trouble, we would change to Plan B and that was I would intubate and Tim would do the IVs. Either way, we would get the job done without delay and no debate would be required.

We also knew that Dr. Lindsay was most likely working or close by, and if we had any hope of getting this man back alive he would try. I had seen Dr. Lindsay save lives before, and he had perfected this science to an art. If anyone was going to be our backup, he was the best we could ask for. I didn't know on arrival that we would find Heather, our very dedicated student, on scene, covered in blood and vomit and doing her best. We could now be a team and this was the best classroom experience she could get.

If anyone could save this stabbing victim, we were up for the challenge. I was going to be responsible for administrating meds once my first job was done and Tim would look after the cardiac monitor after he completed the intubation. We had done so many calls together that we would know where the other one was without even looking. We would sense if the other person was having difficulty just from the change in their voice.

That is what makes a critical care EMS system work. We knew everyone's limitations and when you rolled into an emergency, we were already three steps ahead of everyone else. Today, on arrival, Tim and I looked at each other and shook our heads, as we knew we'd just walked into a complete disaster. Sometimes it's a quiet manageable mess and other days, when everything possible is going wrong, you're just along for the ride.

When we got on scene we decided it would be best to grab our own kits and then we would start our attack. In seconds, we knew we had to go to Plan B, as Plan A was not going to work. The BLS team had a failed airway management situation, with an apneic or non-breathing patient. Heather had to resort to mouth-to-face without a protective one way valve to try to get a seal to ventilate; there was blood everywhere and this was a worst-case scenario. I had been in this predicament before and had done exactly what she did so I knew the reasons why she was doing it, although it wasn't always the best idea. We had a solution and Tim was on it right away.

We always taught our students to use personal protection devices which was gloves, protective eye wear or mask and today that didn't work out so well. It is always recommended to perform mouth to mouth with the proper mask, but when it fails your options are limited. Without a barrier device to stop infection, you would take a chance and do what you had to do. We then deal with the consequences for the next six months, praying we don't catch HIV or Hepatitis B. I had this happen to me twice in my career already and it was stressful and hard but part of the job. A simple needle poke or blood exposure incident can really elevate your stress level!

The patient had no palpable pulse with another attendant doing chest compressions to complete the CPR cycle. The chest compressions looked to be at an adequate rate and depth but it was time for some real ALS intervention.

Tim went for an airway and was suctioning—this was to help clear an obstructed airway—then he would try to enhance the pre-oxygenation and ventilating with a BVM before intubating the patient with an endotracheal tube in the next few seconds. I started one large bore IV and grabbed the adrenalin commonly referred to as epinephrine and started to draw it up in the syringe. Constable Brent Robinson was my IV pole and I got him to start squeezing hard on the IV bag of normal saline to help preload the already empty heart.

We were to administer 1 mg at a time diluted with the typical 9 mLs of normal saline but we had no preloads as they were not available. We had only one 30 cc /mL multi-dose bottle available of adrenalin. I elected to draw up 10 mg of epinephrine in the 10-mL syringe and give the 1 mg or 1 cc and let it then be diluted with the IV fluid running wide open to the patient, thanks to Brent, our human pressure infuser. I knew that next we could try administering an escalating dose of epinephrine, as in this case it could not hurt. We could give the patient a 3 mg or 3 mL dose followed by 5 mg / 5 mL on the following dose. When you've flat-lined, epinephrine is your friend, and in this state any friend that can help is a start. The monitor was on and things did not look good.

I jumped over the patient and inserted a second IV into him and when it was time to give epinephrine, I was shocked. I happened to look across and Brent was still squeezing the life-saving IV fluid, and the syringe that had the epinephrine was slowly injecting itself at the same time. I was going to reach across and inject another dose and this time, I was going to give the patient an additional 3 mLs. I said to everyone involved, "Don't worry about the epinephrine, as God is giving it." I had never again seen anything like this in my life.

The syringe was emptying into the patient very slowly, which defeats the laws of physics. I was almost not surprised, as we needed help from a higher power, so why would I be surprised when we received it?

How the adrenaline was being administered was not possible. It should not have happened the way it did, and when we tried to replicate it after the call we got what we expected. If someone is squeezing the IV bag, the syringe will just fill up every time. It won't empty into the patient on its own at a slow and steady pace. It made for creative charting later but that was the least of our problems.

We elected to transport the patient and make a mad dash for the local ER. The only real chance we had left was in the hands of a trauma doctor.

We had ruled out the common cases of death and we suspected a possible cardiac tamponade. The patient's only chance was Dr. Lindsay and he was ten minutes away waiting for us. Dr. Lindsay was the trauma team leader and we needed to get the patient to him as quickly as possible. Today only a gifted surgeon would save a life for we were just the transport vehicle all while performing chest compressions and ventilations. We also were adding a little lifesaving adrenaline even if it was overrated in the end.

We quickly loaded the patient into our ALS unit and then we looked at each other and decided it was better if we both worked in the back and kept trying to reverse the cardiac arrest. We nominated Brent to drive our unit as Heather and her partner already had a huge mess to clean up. They grabbed their kits and followed us to the nearby hospital. Spending time on scene was not wise as everything that could be done had been done. It was now up to Dr. Lindsay to do his magic. From there on in, everything was a blur in my mind. I yelled at Brent some simple driving instructions. Brent had to abandon his police cruiser and his coworkers and was now one of us. I said simply, "Giver on the straightaway and go easy on the corners." That seemed very clear and to the point.

To this day, I don't remember much about the ride to the hospital, but I do remember rolling into the local ER in Lac la Biche, and Dr. Lindsay was waiting and ready. Brent had used our radio and called ahead and let them know we had treated everything but a cardiac tamponade. We had both wondered if that was the cause of the arrest or if we were just out of life-sustaining blood. In a heartbeat, Dr. Lindsay was cutting the chest open on the left side and if we had a cardiac tamponade, he would find it.

I have never in my life seen such quick and amazing surgical skills. Within no time the pericardial sac was open and we found the knife wound was fatal. The heart was destroyed and not salvageable. This was not our patient anymore; he was now in the hands of the RCMP. Constable Brent Robinson was now in charge, as it was now a homicide.

This one call was great to show that our wisdom had also made some very good call management decisions. With knowledge comes wisdom. With wisdom comes better decision-making ability in EMS. When you become more professional in EMS or in health care, you increase your knowledge and are slowly given more responsibilities, along with respect. With greater responsibility, you are at an increased risk of causing harm to a patient or making a wrong decision.

As an EMR, or a first responder, your skills are limited. As an EMT, your skills are greater but as a paramedic you can save a life—and also harm or kill someone if you make a bad decision or mess up a procedure such as an intubation, or give the wrong drug. Being a paramedic is somewhat like flying a plane. If you make the right decisions, you will have a smooth landing, but if you make mistakes on your approach, you're in trouble.

The basic difference between an EMT and a paramedic is that as an EMT, you can administer eight to twelve common medications but as a paramedic, you can administer about 100. Knowledge is not wisdom. Wisdom comes from time and experience

Over time, we are all challenged and your challenges become more complex as your knowledge grows. You will never stop learning if you are dedicated to your profession and, ultimately, a patient's advocate. I often told my students the following when I taught pharmacology for years:

- With responsibility comes increased liability.
- With responsibility come consequences.
- With increased responsibility come decisions.
- With greater responsibility comes greater liability.
- With greater responsibility come fatal consequences.

Teaching was the one role in my life that I really wanted to excel in for obvious reasons. The first school I taught at was the Alberta Vocational School, commonly referred to as AVC – Lac la Biche. At AVC I was hired to teach the EMT students and helped with the International Life Support (ITLS) course. Then from there I taught the Emergency Medical Responder (EMR) classes, and in 1997 I was hired to be a full-time EMT instructor. From then on, I would be committed to being the best teacher in every class. I would read, study and research as much information to make me better than I was before a question was presented to me. Certain questions would constantly make me research more and more information.

For just over three years I taught many EMR classes and two EMT classes per year, and I finally got to teach my first and only class of paramedic students for Portage College. I started as a regular instructor and by the end I was made the lead instructor. Even today I can tell you about every single student that was in that class. They all had their strengths and weaknesses but together we made a team.

That was the biggest learning curve of my life. It was most likely due to the fact that it was a distance education course and all the learning took place in a virtual classroom. As instructors, we had to learn new technology in addition to addressing our online students' needs. We needed to get our students to master their practical skills so that when we surprised them on a tech week or a site day, they would be able to use them effectively.

152

There are so many factors in emergency medicine that can't be taken for granted and it's hard to teach critical thinking to students or practitioners who are used to following step-by-step guidelines or protocol. But even with all the hurdles we made it work. The fun part was loading our vehicles with equipment and driving to the students around the province to provide them with hands-on education in their own home town. It was sometimes a sixteen-hour day but it was all part of the role we assumed to ensure this province had more ALS members everywhere, and not just in the urban core areas.

My next teaching adventure consisted of teaching the paramedic course in the Community Education Department at Augustana University. This was when I was introduced to intranet education and we took it from its initial trial to being the best anywhere. The classes were dedicated to making our students the leaders in the industry and I'm sure we succeeded on many cases. We were more than eager to make their dreams come true.

Eventually, Augustana had some problems keeping ahead of the changes to the system with an all-too changing and unstable economy. Augustana decided to give up the Camrose Campus and it was consequently taken over by the University of Alberta and we became the U of A – Augustana Campus.

We gained a new president with new ideas and because we were not a degree program, we were basically not a good fit with the university's greater plan. So, we were traded away in 2009 to the Lakeland College Vermillion Campus and overseen by the fire school management. It was a good several years and in 2013 it was over. No more EMS programs in Camrose. I would have to find another school if I wanted to keep helping students become the best they could be with me on their side.

I later became the training officer / paramedic for Beaver EMS. This was a good fit for me for several years. I also taught our local "Give Back" courses and still helped to set up and coordinate the odd

ATLS courses at the U of A, which was also a privilege. I got to help the doctors I had worked with while at the U of A – Stollery in the ER department to teach others to better manage trauma victims.

Many who knew me from my past were very glad to see me. Some were around when I was one of the senior nurses at the U of A – Stollery emergency. They likely had some healthy respect for me as I always treated everyone with the utmost respect, worked very hard and very dedicated to my patients.

My only personal failure as an instructor was my fault. I had agreed to teach some courses for Delta Emergency Training and Matrix Medical College and it didn't go very well. I was teaching our "Give Back" courses as well as some other courses on the side and it cut into their profit and was making it hard for them to get enough students to fill their classes. So, I had to choose between making no money and teaching for fun or for teaching for someone else and I choose the former as it was who I was. Maybe not my wisest choice and to both of my two employers I do feel sorry for the grief I caused you. It was my fault and no one else can take my blame but me.

Another interesting thing I took part in was the creation of the bimonthly quizzes for *Canadian Emergency News* magazine, which eventually became known as *Canadian Paramedic* magazine. I did this for almost fifteen years. We used the current trending emergency medicine perspectives to create our quizzes. Almost every case I used was based on something I had seen or been involved in some way. I always attempted to make the quizzes more of teaching tool instead of an evaluation or an examination tool.

Somewhere after about eighty quizzes, I decided it was time to quit trying to help others when I did not agree with the current direction of our governing body as a whole. It seemed I was fighting the ACP way and it was not my way therefore I stopped writing the quizzes the same day as well as quit all my committee involvements with the ACP. I had hit a wall fighting the ACP's ways and could not ethically travel down a road I didn't want to walk down, so in one day my life changed its path and I headed in another direction. I wanted an EMS world of mentorship as well for us to lead the profession with a more diverse pathway. I knew I had to find a way to help people in a more productive fashion. I wondered if I could somehow create a set of books to change the world. Slowly a dream formed and I started to think of how to change the world one person at a time.

I thought my teaching days were done but then, out of nowhere, Patricia from Keyano College found me and talked me into coming north to Fort McMurray. Patricia knew me well as we had been friends for many years. I had been her teacher, her mentor and, later, her coworker. Together, we attended to a violent murder one scary night. There is no stronger bond then a life and death event between coworkers. We faced a very violent call and we did our best despite a terrible outcome.

That night, we would bear witness to one of the most horrific murders scenes of my career. On the way to the call, we knew it was going to be bad. Patricia reached over and touched my hand and said, "I'm scared." I looked her and said, "Don't worry. I've been to lots of these before." When we got to the scene I took control and we ensured the scene was secured and that if anything could be done it would have been. After we pronounced the victim dead, I did my best to secure the scene. I took digital pictures with the security guard's camera as the RCMP was still about thirty-five minutes away. I was the most experienced person on scene and none of the security personnel had ever seen anything like this before. So, that made me the person in charge until more help arrived.

It was while I was trying to secure the murder scene that a gentleman came in the north door behind us—after I had found a trail of blood heading out the south door, which made me wonder. I said to everyone rather loudly so the man knew I was in charge, "Everyone who is here stays here, and no one comes in or out until the police arrive." This man who had just came into the ATCO Trailer, which was also our bunk house or sleeping quarters with forty-nine rooms per trailer, swore at me, so I told him one more time. He swore at me again and I repeated my message just as he went into his room and closed his door, but with the poor lighting I was not sure exactly which door he went into. I didn't give it too much thought as I had other things on my mind. I thought he was just being a big jerk and never dreamed he was maybe a real psychopath or possibly a cold-blooded murderer.

I would never have expected to argue with the murderer in the hallway after we arrived. I would have thought if you killed someone, you would be long gone I figured they would be halfway to Fort McMurray already. So, to find out he came in the door behind us while we were securing the scene and obviously thought he could get away with it was very disturbing. It was due to my description of our argument that security and the RCMP would open his door and immediately arrest him as the person who had murdered someone without remorse or even a reason.

In the debriefing, later that day I was asked why I went through the door into the crime scene before Patricia, and my answer was simple and to the point. I said, "I can stop more bullets then she can." She is only a little over 110 pounds and all heart. I was made up of 270 pounds of stubborn, dedicated man. I would die fighting and I would not turn my back on my partner. They thought my response was not very funny but I was dead serious. If I died saving my partner, then it was okay with me. Heck, I could not have asked for a better lady on earth to work with so it was worth the risk to me.

In the spring of 2016, Keyano College asked me to build an EMR program that would comply with the new 2017 ACP requirements. Patricia had told them I was the right person for the job. The last time I designed an EMR course on my own was in 1999 for Augustana University. I was more than happy to take on the challenge and was excited to make the course the best of any province. It was to be a sixteen-week course with much more content then the current courses out there. It was a win-win for our practitioners.

I had big ideas and I had a vision, so the rest was easy. I started building it right away. Then Patricia's world became hell for her and her husband, Allan, who is also an EMT and firefighter. The city of Fort McMurray would be tested in a way that no one could have anticipated. The fire just outside the city that was thought to be nothing, waged a relentless attack against the city that went on for days and days, as it tried its best to destroy the city and the people trying to protect it.

The only thing that really prevented us from getting our EMR course up and running for the fall of 2016 was that fire. For days, the Fort McMurray "wildfire" continued its assault and almost burned down Fort McMurray and everything around it. The world responded. Firefighters from everywhere showed up to fight it. They fought the beast as a team and they won.

The RCMP from the surrounding provinces descended on Fort McMurray in droves and made sure that people were evacuated and stayed away until it was safe. It was a form of martial law but without any riots or big fights to fight. The city was evacuated in hours and all of its citizens had to find somewhere else to live for several months. Some lost everything and some lost nothing, structurally.

It was a miracle that no lives were lost with the evacuation. But the bigger miracle was that the world came together to support Fort McMurray. After the flames were out, they started the cleanup phase and then the rebuilding phase, which will take several more years to complete. Keyano, my new employer, was able to save the school building but damage was extensive and it took months before the school could reopen. We instructors had to sit by and wait and I was praying that our dream of getting all the EMS programs up and running was still possible.

Once the school reopened, Patricia and I got our new EMR course ready to finalize. As I write this, we are just doing some fine-tuning and hope to have it running in early 2017. The coolest part was my daughter, Robyn, decided to register as an EMT student at Keyano and started there in the fall of 2016. In no time, she became an all-star student with the marks to prove it. One day I even got to give her EMT class a lecture on X-ray / CT interpretation. It was an amazing afternoon.

Looking back to my Lakeland teaching years I introduced pet therapy to my students. I often took my golden retrievers to class and they went from student to student looking for love. I told management they were drug dogs, but I'm sure they knew they weren't. Every one of my hundreds of students got to know my golden retrievers by name. The day I lost BamBam in a bad accident I was a mess. Bambam was hit by a semi-trailer when his wide load hit him into the ditch while we were building a fence.

The trucker didn't care that he'd hit my dog; he didn't even slow down. I ran to BamBam and was devastated beyond words. I could not save him. No one could. He was trying to get up and come to me, as I was his best friend. He always watched out for me. He was too broken and mangled to get up but he tried anyway. I ran to the house and grabbed my rifle and, while crying, I stopped his pain but not mine. That was one of the hardest things I ever had to do but it was the only thing I could do in that moment.

I was in shock and set my rifle down and I gave him a hug and just held him for a bit. Then I picked him up and carried him to my truck parked in the driveway. I took him for his last truck ride. He loved to ride in the truck and smiled every time he could make a trip anywhere in a vehicle. I called the kids to come home right away. When the kids arrived, we said our goodbyes. Then, as a family, we dug his grave and said a prayer over him and his new cross.

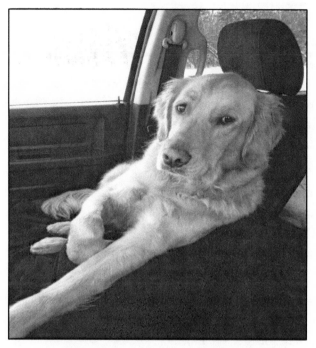

*"BamBam" "Bambam was a true hero." One of
the best golden retrievers in the world."*

The next day I was scheduled to help teach a class of paramedic students and my boss gave me the day off. Pebbles had lost her best friend, who had been her companion 24/7. She was lost without him. We could not stay home that day as it was too sad to sit around. The only thing I could do was take Pebbles to school, so we went and hung out with the students. They were a great support to me that day but, more than anything, they showed Pebbles so much love. They were our family and, after the loss, we needed our family even more.

Thinking back, when my kids were about six and seven, I took them to school on the weekend as they were bored. So, Robyn, who was six, and little Evan, who was seven, started practicing IVs. I was busy with my online courses, marking assignments and preparing for the next class, so I wasn't really paying attention to them. A few hours went by and I went to see what kind of trouble they had gotten themselves into. "Well," Robyn said, "we did some IV practice." I looked and saw they had emptied three boxes of Angiocaths. That's 150 separate IV starts on the IV practice mannequins. I said, "You're going to get me fired," and Robyn replied, "But, Dad, we had fun," and smiled, looking right into my eyes. I was already beaten before I started. I looked back into her eyes and said okay. I'm sure it was worth getting fired when Debbie finds out.

My biggest and only regret from back then is that I didn't do more with my students, but looking back I did my best. One of the ultimate rewards from my colleagues and coworkers was to be nominated for the Alberta College of Paramedics' Award of Excellence and win the award in 2014. This will always be a highlight in my career and to know that so many people were on my side makes me even prouder.

In 2011 while working at the University of Alberta Hospital – Stollery, I was also nominated and won an award after I was recognized by the RCPS Emergency Medicine Residency Program for my contribution toward helping the residents. It was the Emergency Medicine Award for Allied Health Professionals, which I was most honoured to receive.

I know I will always be a teacher as long as I'm still alive. So, in the end my learning will never end. I just hope I can make it fun and help the students learn the easy way. I always thought if you're laughing and learning it can't be work. Many pieces of wisdom I have put together come from the greatest people in the world. When you get a chance to attend any course take it.

As we come to the end of this chapter of my life I can't forget the people who have shared their wisdom with me. I want to thank my great mentors and teachers, including Dr. Mary Stephens, who maintains such a high standard in the ATLS program, along with Dr. Broad who has shared so much with me over the years. Thanks also goes to Cathy Falconer who helps coordinate our Edmonton ATLS programs. You're an amazing, caring lady sent straight from heaven.

Dr. Damian Paton-Gay, you will always be my hero for maintaining such a high ICU and critical care standard and I will always remember our night of hell together. That night we helped save seven kids who had been involved in a horrific rollover. Thanks to the staff at Edmonton EMS, Edmonton Police Service (EPS), the OR staff, PICU Staff and especially the staff in our ER, we as a team of one beat the angel of death that night and kicked her out the front door. It was one of my most stressful but overall most rewarding shifts. We never would have had a chance without everyone being part of the team.

In closing, I want to share some personal wisdom that to this day reminds me that we can learn so much just by listening and not judging others for their lifestyle. I was working one night and we had been running a code for about four hours on a crystal meth overdose. The patient came in with a temperature around 43.6 C and was baking his own crystals all over again. His body didn't want to live but his soul wasn't dying anytime soon, either. I had never seen such a complex situation. It was my first time seeing a paralytic being administered while doing chest compressions, at least in theory, stop the baking process.

The effort by the staff that day to save this patient despite his life choices was so refreshing. The unjudging staff working as a team: our ER docs were amazing, as were the respiratory therapists (RTs) we worked with on every shift. Then along came a blindingly brilliant teacher, educator, mentor and pure gentleman. Dr. Peter Brindley walked in and took over the situation and gave me the best advice I'd ever heard in my life. It works for every patient I ever had that had made an unwise choice in their life. I have made many, so I'm part of this group, as well.

He said simply, "I can't condemn his way of life but it's not conducive to living." We should all take home an important lesson from him. If we can just leave our ego at the door, we can all be part of the team; it's being part of a team that makes us winners in life.

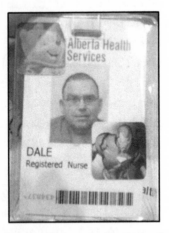

*"Making it right, one patient at a time."*

# "Not Always Easy"

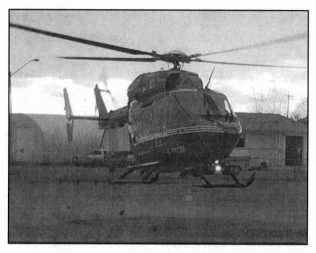

*"Up and Away"*

The challenges of flight medicine are uniquely different than any-thing I ever saw while working on ground ambulances. You have a much more unforgiving atmosphere—literally—and your options for backup are limited and far from helping you, other than by telephone or radio in many cases.

Over the years, I grew more and more comfortable with using air ambulance services as it just made sense in many situations. A big advantage to using an air ambulance is that it comes and takes your patient, and you don't have to leave your service area, which means your local ambulances stay in their home communities more of the time. However, it's not always practical or an option if the air ambulance can't fly due to bad weather or mechanical issues. This is also true if you have multiple patients and will be obligated to take them to different locations. In the end, every ambulance service has its unique advantages and using air has many benefits, but the complications and errors can be deadly for everyone involved when things goes wrong.

My first ride in a helicopter I paid $100.00 for twelve minutes and it was one of the best rides in my life. The most amazing aspect of it is that you can set down very quickly and the ability to access remote areas greatly improves response times. Many years later, I would do a flight where we dusted the river, and it made me realize why medevac choppers in Vietnam made so many mortal wounds salvageable. With the introduction of medevac choppers in the military, true paramedics were made and we owe them all our thanks and dedication. Paramedics today exists because of the war-time efforts and the push to save lives in ways never thought of in the past.

My biggest pet peeve is that many EMS staff do not use aircraft when it is justified. So many times, the mechanism of injury (MOI) is there and we are aware of the severity of the situation up front. The example I would use is of an eighteen-year-old male being ejected at high speed in a single rollover, one to two hours from a trauma centre by ground. If we did the transport by air it could be so much shorter. If we waited to call medevac until we got on scene, we'd have wasted almost fifteen to twenty minutes of the golden hour already, then we'd still need to assess the patient. Many crews will then extricate the patient and put them in the unit. Then they will try to secure an airway. Then they finally realize they are in trouble. "Too damn late," I would sadly say. Sometimes your golden hour is already gone and you have a very bad outcome in the making. Truth be known, the bad outcome was already predicted at the time of dispatch.

The time to utilize rotary is when you know there is bad trauma from the scene, especially when there are internal chest, abdominal or pelvic injuries. Isolated head injures require a neurosurgeon and an OR that can provide the appropriate surgical capabilities and don't benefit from a delayed transport. There also comes a time, especially in more remote areas, where fixed wing is the best transport option weather permitting, aircraft permitting and as long as there is a receiving hospital available. Nothing is easy and sometimes almost everything is against the patient and against you from the start. Do your best to utilize the resources and backup you have to minimize the patient transport time to the most appropriate location.

Ultimately, you need to decide early, notify early, and cut down the on-scene time and transport time if you are to increase the survival rate where an OR is the best option from the start. Rotary and fixed-wing transport saves lives but will increase the costs, as the price of the plane or the helicopter is a lot higher, and it can increase the risks in the wrong environment. Thankfully, our pilots have a zero-risk policy and only fly when the weather and the aircraft are optimal for flying or they don't fly. Canada and Europe have a very good record and have had few air disasters whereas the USA has had many tragedies for many different reasons. However, even with a good track record, sometimes fate is just against us.

We were dispatched for a single vehicle rollover at 11:48 and away we went. On the basis of the MOI alone, I requested a STARS launch to our scene for obvious reasons. The only real reason we would not need them was if the patient was dead or a trauma code, then their destiny was already decided most of the time. We arrived at 11:55 and saw a vehicle that had lost control at very high speed and then struck the ditch and started rolling, end over end, most likely with a slightly twisted motion, as well.

The vehicle was about one hundred feet from the patient and it was on fire as we drove up. As we approached the patient, we saw that the patient was in already in a decompensated state of shock, gasping for breath with an arm ripped off at the shoulder. The arm wasn't even close to the patient. I never even saw it, but it wasn't my priority. My partner that day was one of the best in the world and particularly good with IVs so I made a plan. Dave would get me an IV. I would stop the bleeding before it was too late, then I would secure an airway. I yelled, "Is there anyone here who is medically trained?" One lady said, "I'm a lifeguard," so I said, "You're my BVM, lady. Come here." I quickly showed her how to ventilate after my first tourniquet was on and tight enough to stop the bleeding from the shoulder stump. After the ventilations were going in, I had to apply the second tourniquet.

Dave had the IV ready in seconds and I was drawing up my RSI drugs, as the patient was clenched and I couldn't get in an OPA. The nasal pharyngeal airway (NPA) was contraindicated due to the likelihood that he had a severe head injury. Being that the lifeguard was pre-oxygenating already with high flow oxygen, when my drugs were ready it was time to capture the airway. I pushed the right medications and waited for them to kick in and I knew I had to get the tube the first time. I would get the tube the first time. Failure wasn't an option.

I was ready to intubate and was lying on my stomach, trying to get a view of the vocal chords, when I realized the problem. The sun was shining right in my eyes and seeing the cords wasn't going to happen today. Plan B was all ready to go. I just said out loud, "I'm doing it blind." I guessed where the tube should go by using some internal landmarks and headed to insert the tube in the right hole.

I knew time was against us as the patient had a head injury and was most likely was hypoxic at a cellular level, so I put the tube in as fast as I could. In seconds the tube was past the vocal chords but I couldn't prove it easily. I stopped the insertion with the endotracheal tube roughly at 22 cm for now. Sounds easy, but I'd had many practice runs in the past and that is the only thing that can make you proficient at intubation.

Then I realized I was lying on my stomach and I couldn't reach the BVM easily. So, it was Plan B again, as I leaned my head forward and ventilated down the ET tube with my lips. I could see his chest rise in time with the lifesaving ventilation and I said, "It's in." I looked over at the lifeguard whom I'd promoted to airway helper and said to her, "Don't try this at home!" I then got her to help ventilate while I secured the endotracheal tube. Then we needed to confirm the ET tube placement. I needed the monitor to do this and it was still in the unit. At least we had the airway and could get the patient some needed oxygen and help him drop his drastic high $CO_2$ levels.

Dave ran to the unit and grabbed the LP-12 and we applied it to monitor the heart rate and $SpO_2$. We could then also could cycle the BP every five minutes. Most important, we checked the end tidal $CO_2$ level right away and it was 35 mmHg, which is perfect. I could have not asked for a better number if I tried. Then we packaged the patient and were off to the unit as quickly as possible. This was while the local fire department staff was setting up a landing zone for STARS and looking for the missing arm. As we loaded the patient, we noticed a grand mal seizure starting.

His blood sugar was normal; oxygenation was 100 percent and $CO_2$ was normal. The BP was good, so it wasn't lack of perfusion. I was thinking hard; I had to try to find what the problem was that was now making him have the seizure. What was I missing? Was it our fault that he was having this seizure? Was it my fault? I had to figure it out fast and stop it if possible. We should have prevented the seizure with our initial medications that we'd used to intubate, but they were wearing off quickly and the seizure told us his brain was unhappy.

Looking back to the events, it was most likely the head injury that was the cause of the seizure. You always need to make sure you're not causing or promoting a seizure with your interventions, though. I grabbed my Versed and injected a healthy dose. Having a seizure with uncontrolled bleeding and a significant head injury is never good. The seizure was aborted. STARS-3 was almost on scene, which was amazing timing. I knew this man needed an OR, a blood bank, a neurosurgeon, a vascular team to assess the possibility of attaching the arm, a CT scanner and more help then we could come up with in the middle of nowhere.

After the seizure, we noticed the patient was harder to ventilate and there was decreased air entry to the affected side missing the arm. We noticed subcutaneous emphysema before the initial chest decompression was even considered, but the patient also had hematomas in the upper chest from the arm and pectoral muscles being ripped out of the chest. We decompressed the left chest with a 14-gauge needle with some improvement of ventilation. We then added a second needle for a chest decompression, but it didn't do much good.

The patient needed to get to the trauma centre for definitive care, which would include a chest tube, but that was beyond our skill on scene. The trauma centre would fix that in no time. We were maintaining normal vital signs and we had no drastic alterations in any of the normal vital signs so we were doing the right things despite the patient's complex issues. So far, we suspected a closed head injury, chest injuries, spinal injuries, pelvic injuries and internal abdominal injuries were most likely. Above all, though, he was alive and that said he still could survive this crash even as broken as he was on our assessment.

He had the best chance of any severe trauma patient and his flight should be manageable as long as he didn't decide to bleed to death before he got to the trauma table. STARS-3 was down beside us at 12:23 and the police and fire had closed the highway off. We had a secure landing zone and STARS-3 was getting a report, while getting ready to perform a hot landing, which means the rotors keep turning, which can decrease the overall time on the ground. This was when it hit me like a hammer.

"Crap," I though. "He needs tranexamic acid (TXA)!" I grabbed it and mixed up a one gram vial of tranexamic acid in lighting speed and started the infusion as we loaded him into the chopper. STARS-3 was wheels up at 12:43 and we had done our job. In no time flat, our patient was airborne and headed to the trauma room where I was once a registered nurse in the ER, as well as a frequent charge nurse over the span of ten years, and some of the best surgeons, doctors and respiratory therapists in the world were awaiting his arrival. I walked over the crew who had helped us and gave the woman who had helped us ventilate a big hug. That was teamwork. We saved a life that was so close to being lost.

Calls like that don't come too often, but this year, this would be my third or fourth call where the use of BLS, ALS and STARS made all the difference. Somedays my luck was just around the corner, but my black cloud was always nearby it seemed.

Looking back over the years I will always be haunted by one call. As a front-line emergency worker, you never expect to do a patient harm or have a bad outcome. Hindsight is a wonderful thing, but it won't save you from the nightmares and nights when sleep and darkness are not your friend at all. I assume the responsibility for my mistakes and have always been straight up with everyone. Therefore, I will lay out the call as it went and, if nothing else, I hope my story will help educate others as to how easily things can go bad despite everyone having the best intentions.

That summer day we were dispatched to a Priority One medevac. They had an unconscious patient who needed to be transported to the city for ICU support and critical care intervention. On arrival, we got the report and then were asked if we could also take a second patient, which was a common request. This was the second mistake already. The first one was when a sixteen-year-old kid said to his friends that he didn't need to stop at a stop sign and wound up striking a truck at high speed. The injured patient was taken to the local hospital. I think everyone thought he was okay.

But looking back, everyone missed the Mechanism of Injury (MOI) and the law of physics involved. We know from ITLS that you can take about 40 g of force in a head-on accident; you can also take about 14 g of force from a rear-end impact; but on lateral impact, you can only take about 4 g of force. Our bodies are not built to sustain this type of injury without serious side effects and many times the outcomes are tragic for the drivers and passengers that take the side impact force. Sometimes bad things happen to good people and this was one of those times.

We were asked to take them both, so I had a look at the patient. He was a big, strong man who was awake but in some moderate respiratory distress. They had just finished inserting a chest tube for a pneumothorax. I had a quick look for the chest tube and it looked not quite right and the X-ray wasn't the best, but this wasn't uncommon. I quickly assessed him: his chest drainage system was a different model then I used to but after close inspection I noted it wasn't bubbling air. In a new chest tube insertion, they would normally bubble and air would be removed from the inner chest space for the lung to re-inflate over a short period in time. I also knew some never bubbled and others would stop bubbling if there were any kinks, plugged chest tubes or if the pneumothorax was resolved, it would also have no airflow.

My next step was to assess the first patient, and after assessing him it was noted he was very stable and would most likely be okay and just needed time for the drugs to wear off that were causing him to be unconscious. That day we had an extra EMT as a ride-along and my EMT partner. Hindsight being what it is, we should have taken the trauma patient and called for a second plane for the initial patient. However, we made the decision to package both and be off for the airport, and in forty-five minutes we would be on the ground and to the ICU and trauma centre in no time at all.

En route to the airport, we had one patient in each ambulance as this was easier for everyone but not for me. We were almost to the airport when the first unit pulled over. The EMT was asking for help. The patient was in trouble and could not breathe on his own anymore. We had to perform an emergency intubation. I was forced to do an RSI to get his oxygen saturation back up to normal range. We also had to get his EtCO2 back down to a safe range of between 35 and 45 mmHg. I had just gotten the airway secured when the EMT called from the other unit.

The other patient had decided it was time to wake up from his extended sleep and needed urgent sedation. I went to the patient and got him sedated quickly and reassessed his airway. We were okay and back to the other patient I went, only to find him having some trouble as the rapid-acting paralytic was already wearing off, so I ended up giving him more medication and also a longer-acting paralytic. I thought for a quick second to call for more help, but it would take a second plane at least one to two hours to get to us if they weren't in the air already on another mission. I didn't have that time to spare on the trauma patient.

The patient needed a trauma centre an hour ago. His golden hour of achieving a higher level of care was long gone. We carried on to the airport, loaded our patient without any more complications, and we were off and flying at our maximum speed with everyone knowing we were in trouble. My heart was troubled to know I was by myself as the only ALS person, even though my partner was a very good EMT. I needed help and I needed it sooner than later. Time was running out and I just knew it was going to get worse and I could not do a damn thing to keep it from getting worse. This day would become hell for more than one person.

During transport, I was very busy as we had to keep assessing both patients and provide the right amount of medication and ensure we were always keeping ahead of the next disaster. On final approach, we were still very busy. Thankfully, we had a second ALS unit already waiting for us and we were handing off our unconscious patient and would be transporting our trauma patient to the awaiting trauma team.

Well, as we landed, we had trouble venting our patient and his oxygenation was getting worse. Internal injuries, bleeding, poor oxygenation and time were against us all. Time had doomed him from the start by being in the wrong place when the other truck hit his most vulnerable side. Then over time, the secondary cellular injury occurs and the triad of badness that follows is deadly.

I kept reassessing the endotracheal tube and ensuring I had covered the acronym DOPE, which stands for (D - Displacement of Endotracheal tube, O - Obstruction, P - Pneumothorax or E - Equipment failure). This acronym helped you remember the most common complications with any intubated patient. Displacement of the endotracheal tube—nope, it looked to be at the right depth. It was misting and the end tracheal $CO_2$ level was in the right range but higher then I would expect and I was trying to see what would be the most likely cause. The tube was not plugged, we had a pneumothorax already, but the air entry was sounding on both sides. It seemed as if we also had a flail chest as well as significant chest deformity, and I was not happy with the non-bubbling chest tube from the start of the call.

Using a BVM as the ventilator was not as reliable in any trauma situation. I needed a chest surgeon at my side or, better yet, a trauma team. But they weren't there and I had doomed my patient right from the start for reasons that I could not change. Wheels down, and then we were taxiing to the awaiting units. Help was seconds away but time had already run out.

After getting the patient into the unit, he was decompensating fast. I wondered if he had a massive hemopneumothorax, which is so common in a flail chest and with the impact he sustained that was most likely. After we started lights-and-siren for the trauma centre we lost his pulse. We started the code from hell. We couldn't ventilate and we couldn't decompress his chest with a needle decompression as, even though we carried the correct-sized needle, they were about two inches too short.

I knew what the problem was most likely, and still we could not fix it that terrible day. We needed a chest tube and a blood bank. We had neither. I tried adjusting or milking the chest tube. It was in to the proper depth but would not drain anything. We were doing CPR for nothing, for when you have a mechanical obstruction such as a tension pneumothorax with a massive hemothorax, once your patient arrested, he or she was dead. Our only hope was the trauma team.

We rolled into the trauma centre, CPR in progress, no pulse with chest compressions which could have also been from a massive hemothorax, but regardless with what it could have been we were helpless to fix it. The trauma team quickly took over: chest tubes were inserted and CPR was continued. Within a few minutes, there was a slight improvement. There was a pulse with CPR. Then the patient's pulse weakened. Sadly, it was found the chest tube was not sitting in the correct place, and along with the massive hemothorax and severe internal bleeding, the patient's outcome was fatal due the down time with no pulse, even with CPR.

Shortly after we left emergency, the patient was pronounced dead. He could not fight a losing battle and, ultimately, all his systems failed in spite of our valiant attempt to keep him alive. Despite our efforts, we were in over our heads as we needed to perform much more than we were capable of that day. We needed a miracle that didn't exist. We needed help that wasn't coming until it was too late.

This was one call that when you look back, you realize you were doomed form the start. The trauma surgeon said if we'd had a four-inch needle, we could have decompressed his chest as he was a large man. Without it, we had no hope. We packed up our stuff and left in complete disgust. This death was so tragic to all of us. The accident was preventable. The complications were predictable but in hindsight nothing was going to change the outcome. An early blood transfusion, maybe, but when the bleeding cascade fails the outcome is the same. This call was a worst-case scenario. The angel of death got him and we lost.

Had we been flying with one of our regular doctors that day, it would have likely changed the outcome, but this is the reality of flying to remote locations. You can't always predict the outcomes, predict the injuries, and you don't have a lab and X-ray to your disposal. Once you close the hatch doors, you make do the best you can with your crew and what equipment you have in your plane. You do everything in your power to beat death. Losing a patient is never an option. But we lost that day.

I've reflected on this call at least one hundred times and I still feel responsible. I still think I had the chance to change destiny, but I missed the clues. If we had only had one patient, it would have been so much better; then my complete attention would have been on one critical care patient and not two. You can only manage so much and do so much and we all have a breaking point. I think I broke during that call, but not sure when or how I let it happen. After that day, I learned some valuable lessons but it would not bring back the patient.

A new drug we carry now might have helped. It's called tranexamic acid, or just TXA. It stops or slows severe bleeding but, more important, it slows the swelling and inflammatory response, thus there is less cellular or tissue damage. One gram over ten minutes might have been the miracle we needed, but it wasn't even available for years to come. Also, over the years, we've learned about decreasing tidal volume as it decreases the abrupt intrathoracic pressures which will increase the pneumothorax as well as create a tension pneumothorax, after which cardiac arrest follows immediately.

The best treatment for a tension pneumothorax is a chest tube that must be the right size and must also be inserted into the right plural space. The plural cavity has a fibrous lining surrounding the lung tissue and needs to be ruptured for the chest tube to be inserted to help the lungs to re-inflate. The second-best treatment is a big Angiocath inserted between the second or third midclavicular spaces at ninety degrees.

We commonly use a 14-gauge needle and in the average adult, a 10-gauge is even better. The size of the patient dictates the length of the needle. As in this case, most services only carried only a 1.75-inch needles at the time. But in a larger person you could really use up to a 4-inch. The one we normally carry I love; it is a 10-gauge needle and its needles are 5.25 inches in length. You can decompress anyone with that needle. I've seen as many as 5 14-gauge needles used to help decrease a bad pneumothorax. Just think, the bigger the hole in the lung, the faster the air leaks out. You need to provide an easy way for the bad air to get out of the wrong side of the lung so it can re-inflate. With this needle at my disposal, I hope I will never have another person die from a tension pneumothorax.

A needle decompression commonly just resolves the tension pneumothorax and won't resolve the pneumothorax. These patients need to be ventilated very slowly as if the air is pushed out through the hole quickly, it actually makes your patient worse. You hope to never see a tension pneumothorax on X-ray. If your patient is decompensating quickly and you see the hallmark signs of a tension, you should needle decompress with a needle and arrange a chest tube insertion by properly trained staff. Ideally, a bad trauma patient would get bilateral chest tubes on arrival, especially if they are decompensating or already in a traumatic arrest.

With the arrival and use of Fast Scan portable ultrasound technology, we can identify a tension pneumothorax, cardiac tamponade, or uncontrolled internal bleeding. Just know a patient frequently has a blood loss component such as a hemopneumothorax and this will require TXA and blood as soon as possible in many cases. Chest injuries are never easy to deal with and earlier consult with a thoracic surgeon or trauma team is very helpful if it can be arranged.

The unique challenges of flight are mostly related to the stability of the patient. The more stable you can make them, the better you can ensure the flight will be uneventful. Unlike a ground crew, you can't perform skills on the side of the highway or pull over and ensure the skills are done correctly. In flight, once you close the hatch door and leave the ground, your ability to hear and prevent undo complications are limited.

After arrival on scene, you would always ensure the airway was adequate, ventilation was optimal, IV access was established and reliable, cardiac monitoring or monitoring capabilities were applied and that you were happy with the results. Nothing is taken for granted. It can take sometimes thirty to sixty minutes on a scene call to ensure you're ready to fly, either fixed wing or rotary, with any patient who has complex medical events or major trauma patients.

One of the calls that really made me appreciate the Alberta Air Ambulance program was a STARS intercept on an inter-hospital transfer gone badly. The pharmacology used that day and the administration skills were a unique challenge that many will never forget. Even if the STARS crew played a practical joke on me, it was something I won't forget for the rest of my life. We had picked up a sick person from a local ER and we were to transport him to the city. His situation and the story told me in seconds this call was heading south on a northbound train, you could say. I asked one of the nurses for some extra pharmacology drugs for the trip—drugs that we never carried but should have in this case, as I was never one to be unprepared. I also asked for a 250-ml mini- bag of D5W and put it into my other pocket. Then we were off to our waiting ambulance, which was an old mechanical backup that day but it could fly if needed. I was thinking that this call was not going to go well unless we got ahead of the illness trying to kill our patient. I just wasn't ready or willing to proclaim a defeat, as his family was so worried and praying for him to live.

With the little extra pharmacology, I'd received from one of my loyal and dedicated nursing friends, I was going to win this battle, even if it maybe broke a few rules. I was used to Dr. Palmas' Millennium Medical Control Guidelines, and they provided us with much more flexible guidelines for critical care. Now I was ready and waiting for the hell that was coming right at us.

As we rolled out the ambulance door and headed toward the city hospital, I got my partner to radio ahead and get us backup to meet us in the middle. I knew the backup paramedic as he was one of my past students. In no time, we met at our favorite meeting spot and had a little conference. We came up with a great plan. Dan, my past paramedic student and now my supervisor, said, "Dale let's just do everything right here and get STARS to come to the party and then we can get this transfer heading the right direction." I said, "That's a great idea." We talked about our options and we made sure our EMT partners were on board and they also called the local fire department to get us a landing zone.

I next reached into my pocket for the pressor medication that would and could save a life today. I also grabbed the mini-bag out of the other pocket, as I was set to make a norepinephrine - Levophed® infusion for a peripheral line. A central line was preferred, but today we had run out of extra options so we would take what we had. Any IV was a good start and two IVs were always better than one. We had Dave, my IV hero, as our backup EMT so it was already being inserted without even asking. Dave was always the best person to start an IV, and if he had trouble, it was mine to do and I was more than willing to do it if needed, as that was my nursing specialty.

In no time, I had a norepinephrine infusion mixed and running. I augmented it with dopamine and together we started our battle. We had declared war on septic shock and I knew we would lose with just dopamine, so I had packed some of my personal medication to make our attack more successful. With sepsis and tachycardia as well as low BP, we needed a powerful medication that could get a pulse out of a rock.

The BP was someplace around 60/20, which in terms of stable wasn't even close. This patient I knew right from the start was a septic patient and if he was to live it was going to be a medication battle. We had to perform an intubation as soon as we got the BP up to a safer range, as well as get the cells to absorb some vital oxygen from our preoxygenation therapy, as the levels sucked before due to the distributive shock state.

Dr. Brindley would have been so proud of me as I had the preload of epinephrine and the preload of atropine already set beside him. Then, when we were intubating him, if he decompensated, it would only be for seconds. I would have loved to have had a pocket pressor such as ephedrine, as well, and I can't actually say why I didn't have it—if I forgot to bring it or ask for it, or what. It would have been a good extra pocket medication to have for sure, but I was only human and couldn't think of everything.

We had the airway stabilized and the two separate IV pressors were running well and STARS was still inbound. It was about then I realized that the inverter quit and our IV pumps were dying. So, in a flash, I pulled out my phone and brought up the drip calculation program from the Informed Critical Care – ACLS app on my phone. I had to maintain the lifesaving infusions, as without them the patient would crash as the BP was only being maintained with them both. In no time, we were back in business. I was eyeballing the infusions with a macro-bore 20 drop set, which wasn't a great idea, but when you're fighting a death battle it's an option. You always needed a Plan B in our line of work and I was always trying to ensure I was three steps ahead of the badness. In no time, STARS was on final circle and that was going to save the day. I was really happy to see them coming. As soon as they took over our patient, we could be back in service.

After they landed they came over to the back of our unit. One of them opened the back door and took one look and then said "Shit, it's Dale." They slammed the back door of our unit and then started walking back the helicopter. I said to everyone in the back of the unit "What did I do?" They walked partway back to the helicopter and then turned around and came back. They opened the door and said to me, smiling, that they were just playing a joke on us. Then I proceeded to give them a quick summary and they quickly joined the party.

They looked around and saw I was still eyeballing the Levophed and dopamine infusions and I told them we lost inverter power. Seeing as this was the old mechanical backup unit today, we had catastrophic electrical failure on our emergency call. My luck was holding out as our normal good unit was getting its normal service done today. They both looked at me and laughed. Then someone said to me, "Only you Dale...only you." I said I had no choice and I wasn't losing this battle without a fight. So far, our patient was winning his sepsis battle. It was the ultimate battle of his life and we were on his side. In no time, he was loaded into their aircraft and, skids up, they were off to a city ICU and we had all done a good job regardless of a few extra hurdles on the call.

On arrival, back at our Tofield base, I was asked what had happened as it was supposed to be just a routine transport by ground. What started as a simple ALS booked transport went to hell in a hurry at no fault of ours. I told the manager I had started a Levophed and also a dopamine infusions and he was puzzled. He said, "We don't carry Levophed and never have." I said I had it. He said, "Where did you get it from?" I said, "My pocket." He said, "What?" So, I proceeded to explain myself and he just shook his head and knew I was just doing the right thing even it wasn't regular protocol.

I would likely get some flak from our regional medical director on our audits, but I wasn't going to lose any sleep over it. I was already playing by the critical care rules so I was covered, even if they tried to get me on a deviation of protocol concern. On the other hand, I had an ace up my sleeve. I always had one and used it every time I needed it. I had called #4567, which is the direct line to the STARS link centre at the start of our transport, and they knew our story inside out. They put me in touch with the doctor on call for STARS any time I wanted and I was not shy and would call frequently and ensure we were on the right track in our treatment options.

The doctors knew me well form the University of Alberta Hospital - Stollery and whatever we needed to do was authorized with a thank-you to go. The only thing I could not do was initiate the mandatory IV antibiotics. They would administer the lifesaving antibiotics ASAP on ICU admission. Today we had won and defeated the septic mortality statistics, which were that from 35 per cent to 50 per cent of septic patients died as they were not treated fast enough. My golden rule was upheld today and I will share it with you all as it says what I've always felt is my main reason or purpose in life which is helping patients. It simply says that:

> *"Sometimes we need to bend the rules to save a life, but we should not break our moral code, destroy our ethics, or lose our soul along the way."*

# "Saving Lives"

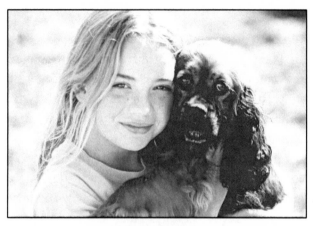

***Abi—"People Who Matter"***

Over the years, I can honestly tell you that the ALS practitioner makes a significant difference in saving lives when utilized at the right time and place. We all help save lives in many cases as long as we ensure our BLS skills are not forgotten. The ALS equipment is only part of what makes the Advanced Life Support (ALS) system work. The most important part is the knowledge and skill set of the ALS practitioner. All levels of care have a unique purpose in every system. As the system evolves, it can become more complex. We all need to do our job and ensure we work to a maximum level to help sustain life at all levels. The EMS system requires the use of BLS, ALS and Critical Care to have a complete and effective system.

The best paramedics I know are the ones who are humble, dedicated to their profession, educated, and will stand up for patients as well as their partners when needed. You need to always be aware of your limitations and know when to call for help or transport to the most appropriate facility. Not every patient fits into a single protocol and never will a single protocol fix every patient. We must be flexible and be ready to work under multiple restraints under the current EMS structure.

When the day comes and you wonder if ALS or BLS is the most appropriate service, think about the severity of the condition. If you're really unwell or unstable and have severe respiratory distress, perhaps decompensating shock, severe anaphylaxis, severe burns, or major fractures and need help, who do you want to save you? I don't want the EMR or the EMT to cancel ALS, I want them to come save my life. Who do you want at your side when you get into trouble? That's right, the person with the most education and the most practical skills in the business. You would want me at your side, I guarantee, if you knew me. I'd choose my friends like Tim Essington. Heather Verbaas, Cheryl Cameron, Tanya Blades and Len Stelmaschuk any day, and if I didn't make it with their help, I'd be okay with that. At least I would know I had the best fighting for me and the circumstances were just against me. Death isn't the worst thing that can happen to us all.

One of the most important lessons I would learn and then strive so hard to teach is that teamwork is always mandatory. When we come across the sick or severely injured, that patient deserves the best ALS care possible. This is not the time for the BLS to attend to the patient; he or she, being the person with the least training, should be promoted to be the driver on that day. It is also a great idea to grab a third attendant if possible to ensure you can do as much for the patient as you can while in transport. This greatly cuts down our scene times, which can result in additional complications or decrease successful outcomes. If you have an airway obstruction, you must fix it right away when you come across it or the patient will die regardless of how much time is spent on scene.

Sometimes your patient needs to be in a critical care support centre such as an Intensive Care Unit (ICU) or in the Coronary Care Unit (CCU) to keep them alive. Some patients need to be close to a blood bank or may need to go directly to the operating room (OR). In such a case, you must get off the scene as fast as possible. Do what has to be done on scene and the rest can be done during the rapid transport to the appropriate location. Always head to the most appropriate location if it's within a reasonable distance; if not, you'll need to just transport your patient to the closest hospital. Regardless of where you are taking them, make sure to call ahead so they can be prepared for your arrival. Communication is the key to the success or the failure of every system.

The EMS profession is only going to survive if the teams work together and as hard as required as well as they must provide the highest caliber of care possible. The BLS and ALS team members must work together for the system to function and thus provide the most efficient ALS care possible. Sadly, this wasn't and isn't always the case in many cases or past situations I've seen as a nurse / paramedic. Over my long career, it wasn't uncommon to see EMRs who thought they were fully capable but didn't even know how to drive a car—never mind a large fire truck or an ambulance module unit that has duals and a diesel engine. I'd see EMTs reluctant to utilize ALS or even call for critical care backup until it was too late. I've seen paramedics bring very sick patients into the ER in a wheelchair and these patients would be in cardiac arrest within minutes with no interventions done on them even when the patient clearly looked unwell and had a huge past medical history. Complacency or a poor attitude kills patients at all levels of care.

In the past, even the lowest-level EMRs were expected to drive an emergency vehicle at high speed with little or no training. This is changing as I write this in order to ensure that all drivers are fully trained. We must ensure we always work at being a more responsible profession.

The problem with new drivers is that they often throw the attendant all over the place until they learn how to drive fast while keeping everyone standing up or safe in the back while working on patients. The test I like to use to test their driving skills is the "fishbowl" test. You take a big container of water and place it on a simulated patient's abdomen. Add some ice in it for effect. If the driver brakes hard, turns hard or drives without undue care, someone gets wet.

It's not easy to drive a big unit as they handle so much differently than a car. It makes me upset if I keep getting thrown around in the back of the unit for no reason other than the fact that the driver has been improperly trained. If I'm trying to stand up and tend to my patient all while they keep braking or accelerating or taking turns at the wrong speed I get hurt. Several times I have smashed my head or face on the safety bar or landed upside down in the EMT saver net all while the driver has no clue I exist. Drive smart and not hard, I would say. You must always drive safely and defensively. Brakes are for emergency driving and not comfort while driving a mobile intensive care unit.

Over my many years of working, I've run into many staff members with poor attitudes. An example of this is that I would often see EMTs who thought they were gods and smarter than every nurse, and even smarter than most doctors as well. This arrogance commonly resulted in sad and tragic outcomes as they would not utilize ALS backup at the right time, and after a kid goes into cardiorespiratory arrest or codes, it's too late to call backup on almost any occasion. I would also see paramedics who had no real desire to help others and just wanted the pay cheque and that's it. They would ignore their patients' suffering as they didn't want to make the effort to help. It doesn't take much for a team to fail but as in every system, sometimes a patient disaster is predictable by teaming up the wrong staff as a team. Ever team has its weakness and its strengths, but putting two bad apples together is just asking for a bad outcome or increased conflict in the patient care.

The worst situation I ever came across was a lazy paramedic who said it was the EMT's day to attend to a call. This person just wanted to drive that day so that was what they tried to do, which is very sad. This is the worst recipe for disaster and so many bad outcomes can be linked to lazy and incompetent practitioners at all levels. When we worked as a team it would not matter if the EMR, EMT, paramedic or nurse was attending, they all had the job and it should always be a team effort. Everyone should know their scope of practice and it's expected that you work to that level. When you need additional skills or an expert, these things are just a call away.

When you have a sick patient, it's the person with the highest level of care available who should attend. If you're suspecting a heart attack and your patient is stable, it should always be a team approach that helps improve the patient outcome. Most of our interventions are done on scene including the 12 lead EKG, so when it comes to a short transport time it really doesn't matter as long who is doing what as long as they are working as a team. I've done several of these calls and ended up driving, as during the whole time I was on hold or talking to the critical care doctors while my partner performed the patient care and kept assessing the patient while en route. When the cardiac monitor says it's a heart attack, it's almost always right (although ectopic beat and pericarditis can make the diagnosis suspicious). Learn to use your cardiac monitor early and keep it attached to your patient during the complete patient contact interval. Then if the patient changes or the patient has an evolving acute myocardial infraction or a serous arrhythmia, you will be prepared. Our Physio Control LP 12 or LP 15s are truly amazing in diagnosing an acute heart attack in almost all cases. I only remember two occasions when it was wrong in my career, and that is rare just the same. When it prints the message "***Meets ST Elevation MI Criteria," it should be an ALS call, at least in my books. But in one of the cases I worked on, I was aware that our EMT knew it was heart attack yet the medic still refused to attend to or treat the patient. I would have kicked him out of the unit and called for ALS backup, stat.

This is what is wrong in our present system. If I was his boss, he would be defrocked of his certification and forced to work in another occupation for the rest of his lives. Now we are being dictated that even if it's not an ALS situation, the paramedic must attend all chest pain calls, which is silly. It's so sad that we must have a rule that the paramedic must attend when if the patient always came first, that would not be required. It should always be a team approach, no matter who drives or attends. I hope that someday we take back control of our patient care and the dictatorship or stringent medical oversight is gone. We should not need to be told how and when to do our job.

Not every patient can be treated the same as we must always consider comorbidity factors as well as take into account if a patient is presenting symptoms, has past medical allergies or medication sensitivity concerns. The complex medical information and the medication compliance concerns matter, just as does a patient's past medical history or recent events. Little things such as the last meal or last drink they took, and what it was, along with their immunization history, menstrual cycle, and recent or missed doctor's visits all matter. All these events must be taken into consideration before we attempt to perform interventions. The patient's SAMPLE history can tell a lot of valuable information if it's complete or available. Without the SAMPLE history, it makes coming up with a diagnosis much harder. This routinely happens with our cardiac arrest and unconscious patients and then we are at a complete loss as to what the differential diagnosis might or will be. It is only after knowing the big picture that we can provide safe and accurate BLS and ALS care.

It makes me wonder why the ALS or BLS doesn't work harder to get the right information from the patient history if it's available. Even small specks of information can be valuable. For example, if your patient states they take a needle one or two times a day, this can be for many things, so ask the right questions. "Why do you take the injection?" and "How long have you been on the medication?" are always wise questions to ask. If it is Lovenox® Vs Insulin I want to know sooner then later.

An important question to ask in trauma patients or the elderly is "Are you on any blood thinners?" Find out what they are on and take it with you to the hospital. Then make sure you try to find their medications and bring them to the local ER with the patient. Expiry dates do matter and look at when the medications were filled and see if the amounts left add up to the expected numbers. Missing pills can mean many things as well about compliance concerns.

Many people are non-compliant or forgetful when it comes to medications. Many times, people will tell me they are allergic to a medication but when you ask more information you find out it's just a side effect and not an allergy at all. The common ones I've heard are a headache after nitro, which is expected, and constipation with codeine, which can bung you up so tight your stool may never come out easily. Also, ensure the medication concentrations are the same concentrations, as they may have different concentrations or be of different strengths. Therefore, the patient could be having extra side effects or the medications could not be working at all due to being over-dosed or under-dosed.

These questions should come from the expert on the call but that being said, everyone is human and we all forget simple things for many reasons. So, for me if it's an ALS or BLS call, I have my brain on overdrive and it's working and constantly thinking of differential diagnoses, and even if I'm not attending I'm listening to the patient care and interactions. In the end, I'm always responsible for the patient outcomes and for the care provided just as my partner is responsible for me and the patient at the same time.

Many times, in the past I've talked to rural EMTs who have told me they don't need ALS as they can do so much that they don't need our ALS help. This, to me, is plain stupid. The sad part is our current rural management style in some regions supports this behaviour over and over as they are too damn lazy to get out and help the staff on the call. If I was the mentor or travelling supervisor in my SUV, I would go to the calls and want to help the staff. I want the patient contact as that is the job I signed up for, not just to drive around and look important.

If it's a BLS call it's still an EMS call. I would ensure the BLS staff were always doing what was right and not just following protocol. Listen to the whole story, then provide suggestions or just make sure the care is optimal even if no ALS skills are needed. Many times, rookie BLS staff doesn't know any better, but after you have seen this type of call or the dispatch information a few times, you can always add some new insight. This is why I always love working with an energetic new staff member. I want to share my wisdom and see that the right care is given in every case.

Over the years, I have heard many nightmares broadcast over the radio including pediatric codes, high-speed collisions involving multiple vehicles, shootings and stabbings when the ALS crews were stood down and not used. Even worse, I've see BLS staff call for help and the ALS attendant go to the scene and not do anything as they simply don't feel like attending. I'd fire them and demote them to an EMR on the spot. Broken femurs, dislocated hips, ejected passengers, unconscious patients…and the ALS supervisor doesn't attend or just follows the crew to the hospital. It still drives me mad.

They should have called in air support or maybe a real ALS crew to take over patient care, I would think.

The ongoing debate by people who are uneducated is that ALS doesn't save lives. Yes, they have a point, but only in a few select cases. If we are called to a situation where a patient needs immediate surgical intervention and time is crucial, transport is mandatory. You then need to consider transport times, transport methods and who can do the transport faster and more efficiently. But you can't start transport or leave the scene if the airway is obstructed or compromised. You can't ignore a pre-arrest patient, which is someone with a poorly maintained airway, ineffective breathing or complications, and especially with severe circulation problems such as profound bradycardia or severe tachycardia and low or very high BP numbers.

You can't ignore the fact that some patients need much more help than you can provide, either. Know your limitations and your scope of practice limitations. Also, know your limitations, just as I did when I had more patients then stretchers and one had a severe airway compromise. I needed to weigh my options and decide what would be best for the patients. If I had stayed on scene and tried to establish a difficult airway, I might have gotten the airway, but I also knew my transport times and the fact that an anesthesiologist could be set up and ready for me on arrival. We need to use our collective minds, our experience and our resources to the best of our ability.

Sometimes being ALS means nothing if the crew is lazy and they don't care or are not prepared to apply themselves. If the ALS crew is lazy and they don't strive to provide excellent care, then in some cases a BLS call would be more appropriate. It is better to provide good BLS and not cause any harm to the patient by performing poor ALS. ALS is more about dedication, knowledge, wisdom and, especially, attitude, than it is about providing care or performing skills just because you can. Just know, all my kids could start IVs, suture, intubate and provide IMs before they were eight years old but they didn't know why they needed to or when they should perform the skill. Never let your job just be a monkey skill or the monkey will do it and you will be out of a job in a hurry.

I had a high school student, Abi, come and take a complete ACLS course just because she was interested. Abi never had the time to read the ACLS book, but she came anyway. I was amazed at how my other students just accepted her and made her part of the team. You see I've known Abi since she was just a baby at the U of A. I knew her when she was a very sick baby. I also knew her dad almost twenty years prior to meeting her when he was my EMT partner in Saskatchewan. It's a small world some days.

When she joined our class, I introduced her and said she was in grade eleven and she said, "Dale, I'm actually only in grade nine." I immediately promoted her to grade eleven on the spot. I thought any kid who would just come to a random ACLS course as a junior high student wanting an extra credit for school deserved the promotion.

If you think we live in a big world, I would say you're wrong. Several years ago, I rescued Abi and her family when their family truck broke down. I was driving through a busy intersection in Wetaskiwin when I noticed a truck just sitting in the intersection and something had to be wrong with it as it wasn't a good place to stop. Other people were just going around them so and I went around the block in order to go back to rescue them. I pulled in front of them and backed up to hook onto them with my tow rope. Then I towed them out of the busy intersection onto a side street. It was minus twenty-five degrees that day with a really cold wind. I then spent several hours fixing their truck and making sure they got home safe as it was a Sunday and the garages were all closed.

Abi's mum said she had seen me before someplace. I jokingly said, "Well, maybe *America's Most Wanted*, as I was hiding out in Canada now. They laughed and then she asked if I had ever work at the

University of Alberta in the Stollery ER. I said, "Only for about ten years," and then she smiled. That was when they recognized me and just like that we were friends for life. She said, "You helped save Abi when she was a baby." It is a small world in health care, especially, and it gets smaller every day.

Abi's medical education started last year, when I received a message from Abi's mum with a strange request. Abi had asked her mum if she could take some medical courses and her mum called me about an ACLS course I was teaching. I said sure, that would be great. In the end, Abi did a practice exam and scored almost 60 per cent, which was amazing, as she didn't know a thing about ECGs or pharmacology before the course. She'd never even read a book on the subject before the course so that should tell you that the power of listening and paying attention really works. It just proves that if you take the time to mentor people in life, anything is possible. If you take the time to actively listen and pay special attention to your surroundings in life, you will learn more than you would think possible. It might even be enough to save a life.

In the past, I had students who were not as successful in my ACLS courses, but it was rare. I've actually failed doctors for scoring less than 50 per cent on a very similar test and they were practicing physicians. So, Abi definitely earned her pass that day and I look forward to seeing her after she reads the ten or fifteen books I gave her after the course was over. In my mind, she was already doing more than some supervisors I had relied on who did nothing for our patients or the lazy BLS and ALS workers I'd seen ignore patients in the past.

Abi wanted to be there and she tried her best and that is all that matters to me. I had won a new friend and in the years to come she will always be a shining light that others can see. Abi will be a future leader for she cares about other people. That's what makes BLS or ALS teams better is people who care about others. If only I could get more BLS services to be like Abi and accept changes instead of ignoring common sense and letting their patients suffer. It would be a great start, but it's going to be a lifelong battle, I'm sure, as most people at the administrative level don't seem to want to make this world a better place. You can't teach wisdom; it's only achieved with time. Abi will receive that wisdom in time as she is willing change, to learn and to participate in her surroundings.

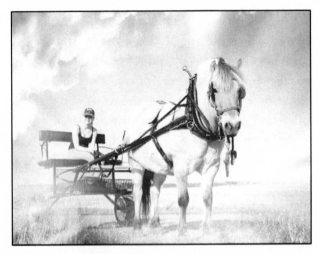

*"Abi proving that life is a meaningful adventure if we just let it be."*

## Chapter 15: Bringing Them Back from the Dead
# "A Miracle in the Making"

There are times when you arrive on scene and just know that your patient is already dead and the time to help them is long past. These are the times we must pay extra attention to the family. Then there are times that you just do not know for sure. I have learned the hard way that you never know when to stop resuscitation as there may be a small chance that they will walk out of the hospital alive. Just when you think they were dead, they suddenly take a breath or their heart starts up after being asystole for a long period and we are all completely shocked. One of the true miracles of EMS is taking a patient who was in complete cardiac arrest and getting them back with a beating heart, breathing on their own and waking up. Then, eventually, they walk out of the hospital. When others may have given up hope and quit, the patients themselves never quit. They want to live and with your excellent care they make that possible.

Over the years, you will see a few of the lucky ones walk out of hospital, but it is rather rare. Always remember that young and healthy equals a better chance at survival, and the older and unhealthier people face increased complications and death in all too many situations. Also, every minute we no pulse we lose at least 10 to 20 per cent viability without chest compressions in a cardiac arrest if we are not doing effective CPR. You need to rapidly decide to work a cardiac arrest or not in mere seconds. Sometimes the deck is stacked against us from the start and sometimes people just have bad luck, so regardless of the effort the outcome is often unchanged from when we started. But if the patient was dead to begin with, you had nothing to lose and everything to gain.

One case that shows me that we need to be aggressive happened many years ago, but it still seems like yesterday. We were called to a stabbing behind the local IGA store in town. I was driving and as I we went past the victim I had to drive around his head to get squeeze into the tight back alley. As I passed him, I noticed the look of death in his eyes. They were open but when it came to brain activity, no one was home. We jumped out and quickly assessed the patient. The story was that he was throwing an empty Magnum wine bottle at the store when it bounced back and it hit him in the chest and he just dropped like a rock. I thought, "It's simple; he's a trauma code and he's dead." He was in cardiac arrest, which likely indicated both respiratory and cardiovascular collapse. One of the deadly dozen was likely our culprit. We needed to see if this was a shockable rhythm, but we had no monitor. We couldn't tell if he was truly dead or this was something we could shock or reverse. We needed to come up with a plan and right now was the time.

In the early days, we had no cardiac monitor in the unit as it was an ambulance used to scoop and run. We needed help, and right now we needed the advanced life support equipment that was in the local hospital if there was any chance for this patient at all. I didn't know it then, but we were going to make a difference in his life and death that day by the quick actions we decided to take. The best shot we had at giving this poor kid a chance was to grab him, put him in the unit while doing good CPR, and get going to the local ER. The first RCMP car arrived right behind us. I quickly told the officer he was our new ambulance driver and my partner and I were then able to do two-man CPR, as it was more effective. We did what was best for the situation.

To me, the best idea was to get the kid to the local ER so he would have a better chance of survival. We got him onto a spine board and moved him to the unit while doing chest compressions. Then we took off like a rocket and in less than a minute we were pulling up to the local ER and rolled into the bay with brakes applied harder than normal. I forgot that the police officer was used to driving tactical but, regardless, we got there in one piece even if it wasn't the smoothest ride.

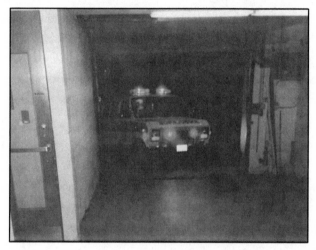

*"Scoop and Run"*

On arrival, the local family physician—who was also ACLS and PALS trained—was more than capable of helping us save a life that day. The rest of the ER staff was ready for us as well. The cardiac monitor was applied right away by a staff member, while others took over doing the lifesaving IV starts; others were helping to maintain the airway and one RN was getting the first round of epinephrine ready to go. It was a well-oiled team that had seen death many times. We had also won many battles on just such cases, when the odds were also not good, by being a good team. As soon as the monitor and defibrillation-pacer pads were on, you could see it was a course ventricle fibrillation (VF) and this was a treatable rhythm. I was thinking it would be a pulseless electrical activity (PEA) or an asystole rhythm as this was most common in thoracic (chest) trauma cases, but not today. I'd seen many similar cases and the patients were dead almost every time. But it looked more like this kid was suffering from commotio cordis. This is rare but very fatal even with a defibrillator present, but it was our only hope.

Despite the good BLS or the ALS care these patients do poorly and the medical community doesn't understand why even today. Commotio cordis typically involves younger patients who are predominantly male; many are healthy athletes who've had a sudden, but blunt, non-penetrating strike to the anterior chest surface. Many receive what appears minor-looking or innocuous-appearing hits that results in the sudden cardiac arrest. The death from ventricular fibrillation tend to come in a very short period and is non-reversible.

Well, we were completely surprised as after just one shock with our defibrillator the patient's heart rate came right back and we had a palpable pulse. This was so amazing, even though there was still a stab wound to the anterior surface of the chest. It looked as if the stab wound was quite superficial and not that serious. Sometimes a stab wound can be somewhat misleading and take us down the wrong differential diagnosis. Looking back, this was such an unfortunate event for the kid but with our quick interventions the outcome was quite good. After all, it sounded as if he had caused the grief to himself, so no one could blame anyone at all.

Many times, working EMS, or in the ER or hospital, we see things that can lead us down the wrong road. Sometimes you think it's one obvious specific problem causing the arrest and you miss the primary problem. An example is ventricular fibrillation from profound hypoxia. We can shock these patients with the defibrillator but unless we revere the original cause of the arrest, they will never do well. Then, despite the treatments we try or the interventions applied the patient does not respond. For us to reverse these devastating outcomes we need to make sure we find the cause early that initialed the arrest and apply the right interventions ASAP.

This sounds easy but it is not that easy in many cases. Even with X-rays, ultrasounds and laboratory results right in front of you, you can miss the original problem. You need to be the detective and dig up all the patient's SAMPLE history or find the clues that tell the rest of the story as soon as possible to change the outcome. If we can get the information it can be the magic key to making the outcome more favourable. Sometimes getting the history is impossible when a patient is unresponsive patients or when they are non-cooperative and this makes our job much harder.

The best way to find the specific cause of a cardiac arrest is to think of the most common causes and then try to rule them out one at a time. There are some common events that initiate a sudden cardiac arrest that we can reverse if treated sooner than later. Drugs such as adrenalin also epinephrine might actually worsen the 30-day outcomes in a cardiac arrest but they are not sure as the 2015 American Heart Association guidelines hinted towards. I truly don't know but we will see in the years to come I'm sure.

We have an acronym, AEIOU-TIPS, which helps some people remember the common concerns. It has been used for years in the EMS and critical care world. There are some really good ways to prevent death when our patients are sick or not responsive and many people have no idea what they are so I will share them with you all just to make you more informed, and the medical people who read this will laugh a little I hope. Sharing this little breakdown of our acronym of AEIOU-TIPS might help you and your family to know when you should seek medical care in a crisis. If I had my way I'd make the Emergency Medical Responders (EMR) course a junior high elective in every school around the world.

**AEIOU-TIPS Explained:** *This is still one of the best and easiest acronyms I know to remember the most common causes for a patient to be altered or unconscious. Try to think of the acronym AEIOU-TIPS and use it to assess patients who are not responding or may have a problem with an altered mental status.*

**AEIOU-TIPS stands for the following:**

A   *Alcohol, Abuse of Substances, or Acidosis*

E   *Epilepsy, Environmental, Electrolyte, Encephalopathy, or Endocrine*

I   *Infection, Meningitis, or Sepsis*

O   *Oxygen Deficit or Toxicity, or Overdose*

U   *Under dose or Uremia*

T   *Trauma (acute brain injury or hypoperfusion of brain)*

I   *Insulin (low or high blood glucose)*

P   *Psychological or Poisons*

S   *Stroke or Shock*

*All of the above information covers some of the most complex issues seen in patients. The sicker the patient is the more complex the issues are and, commonly, the harder they are to reverse and stabilize. Anyone interested in the most common medical concerns should try and read the Advanced Medical Life Support (AMLS) textbook as it is an easy read and very interesting. The more knowledge you accumulate and the more you learn in life, the more you realize that we only know a very limited amount of information. I digress...*

Many years later I would be presented with another sudden cardiac arrest with a very unpredictable outcome. I was sitting at the triage desk when a mum walked up to me and said she had a sick baby. I immediately got her to sit in front of me and I proceeded to take the cover off from around the baby's face. I could see right away that this was not a good situation. I just grabbed the kid out of the car seat and put him on one arm and initiated chest compressions. You could tell by his pale, limp body that he was in cardiac arrest. Apparently, he was okay when she put him in the car seat at home but he was now in full cardiac arrest. I cradled most of him on one arm with his legs dangling at the base of my elbow and his head between several fingers. I quickly ventilated him with mouth-to-mouth ventilations and ran while doing CPR toward the pediatric resuscitation room. When I entered the department, several nurses saw me running and doing CPR at the same time. They knew right away I needed help in the worst possible way. "Code Blue! Code Blue!" I shouted at them.

The staff in the pediatric department knew me very well and they could see I was bringing them the worst trouble you can imagine. They knew exactly what was wrong as they had witnessed many cardiac arrests come through the doors. I was thinking, "Time is muscle, and a pumping muscle saves brain cells," so as long as we had me as a mechanical heartbeat, we had a chance today. Today I was the heartbeat on steroids and I was pushing hard and fast. Nothing would have stopped me from trying my best even if it was too late.

So many times, we would work the kids for up to one or two hours and lose. But sometimes we got them back, only to never get them to live long enough to be discharged. In children and infants, it's almost always an airway issue that causes them to go into cardiac arrest and not related to the heart. The heart quits as the hypoxia shuts it down and it must be reversed to change the overall outcome.

Just remember, in infants and children A+B=C, which is Airway + Breathing = Circulation, in most cases.

All we can do is to ensure that we cover the basics and that we do this in as short a time as possible. The first priority is always to establish rescue breathing and secure a good airway. The respiratory therapists (RTs) and physicians were on that right away. An IV was inserted and a blood sugar test was performed right away. Then we would stretch out a Braslow® Tape beside the infant and it would tell us the correct emergency medication dosages. Also listed were the correct endotracheal tube sizes and the dosage for the infusion medications that could be used. As soon as we got an IV flushed and secured the correct dosage of adrenalin was then infused and circulated with about ninety seconds of CPR followed by a pule check.

This day was a good day as we got a pulse back sooner than expected. It was suspected we had caught the respiratory arrest in time had done the right things right away. This story had a good ending but had the mum not come up to me at the desk looking distressed, I might have let her wait a few more minutes. That day we won but the next day we had almost the same situation and we lost. My working partners told me I could not do triage for a bit after that bad weekend as everyone hated to see kids die and babies were even worse. I was happy to just go work in a pod and forget what had happened the day before. Some days we win and some days we lose.

The most important point to remember is to use our time wisely and try to find the initial cause of the arrest and identify any complications right away. Giving epinephrine will only help if the cause is anaphylaxis or a low-rate complication. A quick review of the patient's SAMPLE history will let you to know your patient's past medical history and last admission report is seconds. Never leave any stone unturned and know that sometimes even with laboratory, X-ray and invasive monitoring, we won't always be able to pinpoint the complication or reverse the outcome. Do your best and work as a team and destiny will declare itself sooner than later. Most days you don't need o wait long for trouble to come your way in health care or in the EMS world.

## Chapter 16: Bringing Them Back Dead
# "Sometimes We Just Lose"

There may come a time in your career when you think you know everything there is to know about keeping people alive. Well, sorry to be the bearer of bad news, but they forgot to tell you about the cases you would lose. There are some types of cases you will lose almost every time. They possibly also forgot to tell you to consider the laws of physics or about the man called "Murphy," along with his laws of bad luck. Something I never really thought about until after working for many years is that you can't beat the law of averages every time. It doesn't matter how good you are or how good your team is, death is always waiting in the wings. So, this chapter is about some of the things I was taught the hard way. We aren't meant to win every time. Sometimes we *will* lose and if we knew the patient would face a long ICU stay and never wake up, we possibly would have stopped trying to save him or her even sooner.

Gibbs' Rule #11 is a good one to keep in mind. It simply states, "*When the job is done, walk away.*" So, after your round with death you need to accept it and know you did your best. Once the outcome is confirmed and the time of death is called then you next job is to look after your team. Do your best to ensure your team members are okay and are not left in a very dark place.

You need to always know your team is safe and not left behind. Sometimes they need you more than words can say. Offering a hand to hold or an ear to listen is needed in some cases more than others.

To know someone cares can give someone a reason to get up and go on when they feel as if they have nothing left. Matt Anderson's song, "When my Angel Gets the Blues," says it so well. The message to me is simple: When we see someone, who is in trouble, we help them. When they are down, we pick them back up. We don't need to know why they are in trouble and they don't need to tell us why. Then once they're up on their feet again, if we can, we need to walk away.

Walking away might sound easy but it's not. When we see, for example, an elderly person who passes away in their sleep, I feel a little relief. I feel that this is a true blessing as they are not suffering or dying a painful death, so it's the best way to go when a person's time is up. Watching cancer patients die in severe pain, or with severe shortness of breath is another story. Some cases are easier than others to let go of in your mind.

Multiple-patient deaths and pediatric deaths were always the hardest for me to forget. Sometimes it can be something unique about the patient or about what happened to them that makes it particularly difficult to let it go. If we didn't feel something, then we would not be normal. The sounds, the smells and the feeling of that awful day can come back when you least expect it.

I would challenge everyone to think about this the next time they are working with a new graduate or a new employee and make sure they understand that it's normal to feel upset or sad. We need to ensure we are a good team and a good team always looks after each other. We should strive to help others in their dying moments and share their suffering and pain, even if just a little. Even a little help can go along way when someone has no one else on their worst day.

As a medic or nurse, when you look around, you see evil lurking everywhere. Somedays I wonder if maybe hell is actually right here on earth. On many calls, we are dispatched to very bad situations and a patient's fate has already been determined before we even arrive on scene. We also see the same severe cases come into the local ER at any time of the day with or without warning. The staff members in the ER are the ones who deserve the credit for doing everything possible to keep a patient alive in so many bad cases. Despite the losing battle they are up against, they put up one hell of a fight over the next few minutes or the next few hours regardless of the expected outcome. They are the real heroes.

One such call I will never forget was when one of our EMS crews was dispatched with the RCMP to a possible crime scene. They came across a very bad event which, thankfully, only involved one patient. Someone had allegedly shot this man point blank with a shotgun and left him to die. The mechanism of injury suggested that his chances of living were almost nil despite the EMS and ER staff's quick and aggressive interventions. Nothing can take away the level of destruction caused by a shotgun blast at point-blank range.

They did everything possible on scene and then loaded him and came directly to us in the ER as fast as possible. If there was a chance for this patient to survive, it was to get him to the closest hospital as quickly as possible. It was mandatory to use our air ambulance teams for longer distance transfers if possible. They sometimes had to stop for few lifesaving interventions but most of the interventions can be and are done en route. Staying and playing on scene is a myth for good EMS staff. Very few crews would waste precious time on scene when the situation was this grave.

Normally the crews will load a patient and perform almost all ALS skills en route. I've intubated at high speed as well as put in 24-gauge IVs in little babies at over eighty miles an hour on several cases. When you need the hospital staff and their life-saving medications, that's where you need to get going, and wasting time on scene won't save lives if you can ventilate or provide good CPR to a patient in cardiac arrest. The local hospital staff can attack a sick patient as a team. If we get the patient back with a pulse or stable enough to be transported out, they can then be flown or taken by an ALS ground crew to the waiting trauma teams.

No two calls are identical or have the same circumstances. We have a blood bank ready and waiting for the major trauma cases which is very helpful in certain cases. We also can use tranexamic acid (TXA) and have it ready at a second's notice. These patients are commonly all in hypovolemic shock, which means they require critical care, surgical care or an ICU in most cases after they are stabilized. The aftercare must be diligent to ensure the outcomes are successful in the severe trauma cases. The whole team approach is the best life-saving approach. Not one part can be missing from the team. From the first responders and the quick actions of the police to the EMS care and ER stabilization and finally the OR to repair the damage followed by a stay in the ICU to overcome unwanted or unforeseen complications, all of these people greatly improve patient outcomes.

The hospital is required for interventions not used in EMS today. The ER has chest tubes and the central lines that major traumas need to have inserted sooner than later to ensure the threats to their lives are stabilized quickly. In serious cases, there are many critical interventions that are required to change the probable outcome from a negative to positive one. That day we got the shotgun victim started like all too many, and as soon as the call came in, we were ready and waiting to fight a hard battle. The atmosphere, when a call like this comes in, changes immediately, and the serious looks and additional adrenalin keeps everyone on their toes.

The patient was rolled into the ER and a Code Blue was called. We brought the shotgun-blast patient to an awaiting trauma team and started the resuscitation. Knowing the mechanism of injury, it was either going to be a very busy day for us or this patient was going to be dead real soon. The emergency doctor can call a cardiac arrest case in a short period of time if he sees that the patient has no chance of living and, especially, if we perform a fast scan of the heart and see no cardiac activity.

This case looked grim right off the bat. The patient's colour was consistent with bleeding out already and the mechanism was the most likely contributing factor. We were doing CPR very well, but poor perfusion and poor ventilation were also a concern. With the shotgun blast, the injury was most likely to be to the liver and the lobes of the right lung which made things even worse. We were preparing for a chest tube on the affected side so that we could insert a central line and pour in the IV fluid and the waiting blood products. Then someone changed our plans and the lights went out for all of us.

The lights literally went out and it was completely dark in the trauma room, as there was no source of natural light. This made it hard for us to do anything, much less cutting into the patient's chest with a scalpel or putting in a central line in the groin. Staff grabbed their phones and we used them for lights for the time being, as we waited for the overhead lights to come back on. Normally, it's almost instantaneous: the generator kicks in in a few seconds. But today that was not the plan. With the sudden blackout and the poor prognosis, I thought maybe someone was trying to tell us something. I said to the whole room, "Maybe God is telling us we should just quit." Then, suddenly, the lights came back on. I'm sure others in the room at the time were thinking the same thing but didn't actually say it. We all did our best that night and more, but in the end, it was declared a homicide as we were unable to save the patient.

In my position, I was supposed to be in charge of the codes throughout the hospital on my shift and I tried always to ensure we were a team. In reality, this was hardly necessary as the ER staff and the doctors I worked with were some of best in the world. I sort of just made suggestions and tried to lighten the mood by making people laugh or smile.

The best one liner I can remember was simple and to the point. It was something my brother had said once and was perhaps a little inappropriate but still funny to me. He said, "They died of natural causes as they fell on my knife nineteen times." Not everyone got it but most of my friends smiled and understood.

We all settled into finishing with our cardiac arrest patient after the lights came on. It was amazing to see a pulse for a few seconds after the chest tube was inserted, only to lose it and soon after it was an asystole arrest. A quick fast scan of the heart and the code was called. Then the RCMP had a case as this was now a homicide and not our problem anymore. Sometimes we win but today it was a lose-lose. The one thing the day did was bring us closer together as a team. We had some new staff on board and it was a good training event as it was also a unique code. It was a trauma code with lots of interventions happening all at once. This is where the new staff can be utilized well with the senior staff to supervise and show them the right way to perform new skills for the first time. Overall, it was still a good code even with the bad outcome. The outcome was predetermined with the shotgun blast. It was just another one of our long nights as a team.

Over the years, I would come across many tragic events. But one of saddest cases I ever had still haunts me, even knowing there was nothing we could have done to help. I had gone home to spend some time with the kids and was going to help at our family farm with sorting horses the next day. We had hooked onto the portable corrals and headed down the road toward Carnduff, Saskatchewan, which is my home town. I had just passed our neighbours, the Norths', farm when I looked out toward the dam and I could see a police car and an ambulance. I couldn't turn around so I just pulled over and pulled the pin and left the corrals on the road. I knew something bad had happened but I hoped I could be of help. The Norths were really good family friends and I'd be damned if I couldn't do everything I could if they were in trouble.

I pulled up beside the ambulance and my little Evan was with me and we walked around the ambulance. That was when I knew it was terrible. The EMS crew was doing CPR on one of the kids. The boys were riding the quads and somehow one of them flipped and landed on top of one of them. The family all knew me but the EMS crew and the RCMP on scene did not. I told them I was a paramedic and I could help. I looked at Nolan on the monitor and it was a "No shock advised," which was what I expected. I asked them as they were a BLS crew if they had an IV kit. They said yes. I told them to get it. I quickly inserted an IV and started it running wide open, and asked if they had another. They got it and I had it inserted and running right away, as well. I wanted to get in a few boluses of 20 mL/kg and at least try to reverse one of the most likely causes of the traumatic arrest. The oxygen and the BVM would be looking after the hypoxia problem, so that was not an issue today.

I needed intubation equipment, I needed blood products and I needed help, but none of it was looking good with a traumatic arrest in the open field so far from a hospital. "Those damn quads," I thought to myself, looking over at them and thinking that they are so useful on farms but so dangerous at the same time. I had seen their traumatic effects on more than one occasion in the past and most often speed or alcohol were the main factors, but today it was just a case of bad luck.

If the cause of the arrest was possibly hypovolemic shock, we could hopefully reverse it enough to get a pulse back with a few litres of fluid. But I still had no idea where the injury was. It could be anything from a severe head injury, to a cervical spine injury or a broken neck. But it was also possible to have a severe chest injury or internal severe abdomen bleeding or even a bad pelvic fracture, all which were very serious.

This poor kid needed my friends from the trauma team and I was in the middle of a damn pasture. They would have helped me in a heartbeat. They all knew what would have helped and we could have attacked this little man and provided him and his family with some hope. We could have changed the outcome if they were with me today. I could only hope and pray that was still possible, but it wasn't meant to be at all.

In no time, I had the two IVs wide open and then I needed epinephrine. I already knew the answer, as they were just a small BLS service, but asked it anyway. The answer was no. I asked the family and the police about an epinephrine or EpiPen and none was present. In a pinch, I could have made it work but we didn't have on anyway. Then the RCMP officer said a second officer was coming with a doctor. I thought about that and wondered if he would bring drugs. If not, we'd be no further ahead.

I thought we should maybe just load him up, do CPR and get going to a hospital. It seemed like our best chance to change the outcome. But Oxbow hospital is about seventeen miles away and CPR in the back of the ambulance isn't always the best; even when we try hard it can be ineffective. So, we just kept doing CPR and waited it out. In no time, the local physician was on scene. When I looked up, I knew it was over when he got out of the car with nothing in his hands. Our family doctor was over eighty years old and was an amazing physician but had no training in advanced life support and this was needed today more than anything. It would be a short and ineffective code without the right people. Without the right medications, we had no hope left. I was lost and no one could help me in this terrible spot I was in. I was helpless but not defeated.

I could have used any one of my good friends to help improve the outcome that day. I'd have given anything for Dr. Sookrum, Dr. Chang, Dr. Sevcik, Dr. Jain, Dr. Ali or any one of the pediatricians from the Stollery to be at my side, but today it was just me. Any of my old nursing staff or our respiratory therapist would have stood toe-to-toe with me and we would have done some amazing work.

We would have moved the heavens and earth to save him. But not today, I thought, it is all over. The angel of death had already declared the ends before we had a chance. In the end, the devastating injury from the quad had done some serious damage and none could change the outcome.

As soon as the doctor set eyes on my neighbour, I knew from the look in his eyes that we were done. It was over when the doctor said to stop CPR and then walked back to the police cruiser. It was like being hit with a big truck. We had lost despite everyone trying what they could. In my mind, we were not done just yet, as there was still one more thing that had to be done. It was the right thing to do. Nothing was stopping this from being my last suggestion as the impromptu leader on the call. Even if I was not licensed in the province, I was leading it anyway. I would deal with the consequences later if it ever came up. I didn't care as I could not change the outcome now but one more feat was required.

I said to the mum, dad, brother and sister, grandpa and grandma, to come over and hold him. I told them to tell him that they loved him and just hold him tight. I knew it was not much but it was the only thing left we could do. This was the right time to show him love and you could see it in their distraught faces. I noticed my brother had arrived and asked him to take poor Evan, who was just standing watching all of this with the police officer. At least he could see his dad try his best even if the outcome was not good.

We stayed out in the field for some time. It was a sacred but special heartbreaking time for everyone. I didn't want to be there as I was completely helpless, but in the end, we all did what we could. The EMS crew was amazing and the local RCMP would and have seen this type of disaster one too many times, I'm sure. They are the true heroes and needed our appreciation as well that day. That call and many more over the years would teach me that it is not just about the terrible loss of the person in the cardiac arrest. It's about everyone involved. This call affected many people both directly and indirectly.

When we look back and learn the outcomes were possibly changed due to other interventions, you can feel hurt and think you maybe you let the team down. I know that it's easy to second-guess results looking back or from the outside, but this is not practical or realistic. Therefore, if you excel in your education and learn from the best you can be the best. If you're the best and do your best you will also know that everything you do is a learning adventure. We will never know it all and after every call I still learn something new. It's then my role to share that knowledge with others and ensure the patients we see in the future receive the best care we can provide.

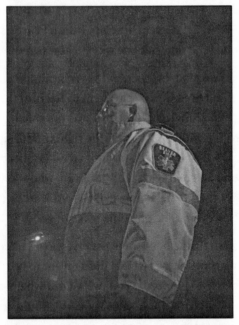

*"Doing what's right is all we can do some days."*

*Chapter 17: Volunteer Firefighter*

# "Close Calls and More"

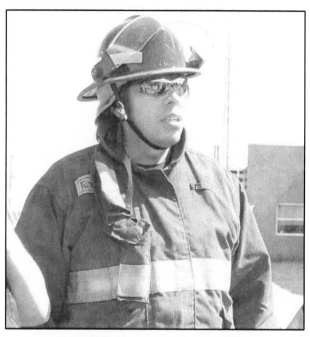

*"Our EMS / Fire Family Matter"*

I always wanted to be a firefighter and I knew if I got the chance I was going to achieve this dream someday. To be a volunteer fire-fighter is a unique challenge and a privilege. We would serve our community 24/7, and without warning your day would sometimes be interrupted. Many times, while others slept, we were fighting fires. Still, responding to MVCs and extricating trapped patients was our primary role.

Sometimes we were called to help with situations that could be very graphic and emotional for many staff; even if they never said as much, these cases affected everyone. We often found ourselves removing deceased people from mangled messes and we would do our best to remove them with 100 percent dignity. In the dry season, we would have fire calls after fire calls without time to rest or to recharge, as there were so many grass fires. We just worked our butts off until all the fires were out. We also responded to smoke alarms and false alarms. If you called, we came as a team.

The closest I ever came to being in trouble was during a normal house fire. About 3:00 a.m., I was awakened by a terrifically loud crack as lighting had hit something close by. It was such a loud bang that it shook the room. In a few minutes, the first alarm was put out on my pager and in no time, it was toned out as a general fire call. All the department members were being called. I was working days as an ER nurse, so my day just got lengthened. Back then it was common to be on call during the weekend you were off and then you were expected to go to all fire calls. During the week, you went when you could and prayed enough firefighters would show up. But on a general call, it was everyone, every time. A general call would ensure we could man all the trucks and, if needed, would attack from all sides to ensure it was the safest and best attack. We all had assigned trucks and assigned captains but we would be given jobs as we arrived on scene by the deputy chief or the chief. My captain was very cool and he would keep us safe and I was never once scared when he was my leader.

After we got to the fire hall, we donned our bunker gear in seconds and, grabbing our jackets and helmets, as we bailed onto a truck and off we went. One or two of the trucks that were able to pump higher amounts would normally grab available hydrants and ensure we always had water, as we would empty our water supply in no time at all. We always had a backup plan on every call that would seem redundant but was essential for our safety just the same. We hadn't had that many close calls so far but every fire could be your last if you weren't thinking, and you always watched out for your family. We were the eyes and ears for our brothers on every call.

On this call, I was assigned to using breathing apparatus and was to be on the inner attack. After one or two bottles of air I had changed out and I was to go in with a senior firefighter named John to do a quick search upstairs for a missing cat. I had put on my new bottle and we were working as fast as we could, searching in the near-black smoke-filled upper level. We still had active fire but it was almost all knocked down. All was well until when I went to take in my next breath it wasn't there. I tried again and nothing. Then I panicked. I nudged John and said, "No air" to him, pulling the mask away from my face enough to inhale the smoky air in the room. I was planning to scramble down the stairs to try to find a way out. The house was filled with smoke and I was panicking. Not being able to breathe wasn't helping my racing mind. It was a pure adrenalin rush that said get out now or die. Fight or flight was the response that was being fed by my brain. Today is not your day to die so get the hell out!

I knew time was against me. I wasn't sure I'd make it but I was going to try anyway. I made the "down" signal and pointed to the staircase and John, the wiser, pointed to the closest second floor window that was the new escape plan instead. It was the closest and the quickest way out of immediate danger. So, I just headed that way and dived head first out the window onto a level roof structure. John was at my side, coming through the window and wasn't leaving me. In seconds, a ladder was beside me and my firefighter brothers were pulling me to safety. In a matter of a minute I was on the ground safe and had my mask off and I was breathing the best air in the world. That was too darn close, I thought to myself. Thank God for my partner, always at my side.

In no time, my scare was over. All that had happened was a little piece of wood had gotten stuck in the regulator when I had changed bottles. Just a fluky problem but scary all the same. It made me appreciate my partner much more than usual. Entering a house for a rapid search is never without risk. Even when a house fire is almost out, there can be concerns that will make your day much worse in seconds. You get to know the real meaning of the word "trust," as you know if your partner gets in trouble or you get in trouble, one of the team will be at your side and get you to safety, or your team member will get you to safety or die trying. You grow a bond that is second to none.

Over the years, I found it so much fun to participate in cross-training and from time to time I would cross over the line and help the other responders in need. One of those calls was a good example of me responding as a firefighter but transporting as paramedic. I was wakened at about 4:00 a.m. for a high-speed crash. It was a general page and everyone was called and slowly everyone arrived at the hall as the roads and weather were terrible. It would do no one any good if we crashed on the way over. In no time, we were off and in less than a minute we came across the disaster. The police were trying to stop another car and it took off at a high rate of speed. Then, as it crested the top of a hill, it became airborne and the flying Mustang had a bad landing. As it came down, its rear end caught and tore right out from under the car. No amount of supercharged Ford power would make it drive fast ever again. On landing, the occupants were ejected and landed in the snow bank. Apparently, they hadn't been wearing their seatbelts, but I guess if you're running from the cops, seatbelts are probably not your first thought. I bet when they were ejected and went face first through the windshield, they had second thoughts about drinking and driving. It was deathly cold out and they were lucky they had a soft landing.

On arrival, I could see one of the local paramedics trying to get his Sp02 machine to register on one of the victims lying in the snow bank. My captain looked over at me and said very clearly, "Dale I think you should take over this call." I did as I was told and the paramedic never even noticed that I took over as he was still lost to the fact that the Sp02 was not working. In no time, we had the patient packaged, loaded and off to the local hospital. The rescue truck came to claim me, and as soon as I helped transfer the patient onto the ER stretcher, I just disappeared. It was less paperwork and I was okay with that. I'm not sure why the paramedic was not awake enough to notice that the cold temperatures would make the Sp02 monitor fail, and unless the patient was in a warm, stable environment, it meant nothing anyway. Scene safety is always a factor and the weather made it a scene hazard so it wasn't a priority to undress the patient or evaluate vital signs out in the ditch anyway. It was a good teaching point I was to ensure I remembered.

The volunteer firefighters got to participate in fun stuff, as well. The coolest thing we ever got to do with the Wetaskiwin Fire Department was to compete in the World Fire Fighter Games in Edmonton in 1996. My partners were Tim Essington, EMT-P, who was from the Wetaskiwin Rescue Group and Bruce Wade, EMT-A/Firefighter, who was also on the Wetaskiwin Fire Department. We were supposed to have a fourth partner but we had no one else so we just made up for it with teamwork. In the end, we were the only team to not lose a member from a scene hazard. When it comes to fire and rescue that means everything. It counts for everything to not lose a partner on a call.

They failed us for not stating that we'd had to call for a transport crew soon enough. Still, we kicked butt and we knew regardless of the oversight we had done well. In the end, we got a bronze medal, but in our hearts, we won the gold.

We responded to many trivial calls, but a few calls were life-changing. The closest I got to be blown to another world was when I was at a structure fire with Wetaskiwin Emergency Medical Services, helping our firefighter partners on scene. I was helping my friends on the Wetaskiwin Fire Department move our support fire hoses and whatever else I could do. I was just in my EMS jump suit without my firefighter gear, so I was not protected from much at all. I had to stay away from any active fire or heat or I would have melted like a marshmallow and it would hurt. The initial attack was still in progress and it looked as if we were going to win. Unbeknownst to any of us, we were about to get the surprise of our life. I was really close to the building and I wasn't worried as the concrete cinder block wall was protecting me, or so I thought. I had just put my head down and went behind the green dumpster when hell came looking for us. I had no idea that I could be saved by a dumpster, but that day it was my saving grace. That was the best green dumpster in the world I tell you. I almost had my birth certificate revoked by fire and flying debris. At least it would have been a quick death, I would hope.

As I went as low as I could to get under the corner of the lid and was ducking behind the dumpster, the building exploded. A tank inside that we were not aware of was heated up and slowly it turned into a time bomb. It would be an explosion seen and felt for miles. I was only a few long strides from the outer building wall. All of a sudden, I could see chunks of the building passing in front of me and the lid from the dumpster deflected the blast over my head. I could have not been in a safer place in that second of time. Mind you, I was about ten to twelve feet from a building that was all of a sudden blown to hell. The loud boom and the force of the explosion was felt next. It was amazing, the feeling of the after-effects, as they it pulled everything behind the initial force. A once-in-a-lifetime event, I hope. My guardian angels were most likely holding the green dumpster to the ground. I should have died or gotten hurt that day, but I was spared.

We got to work and we had two injured or exposed firefighters to deal with who were hurt from the explosion. Even with the proper fire gear and breathing apparatus, they were too close to the explosion. They were hurt and needed us and we were ready for action. We ended up transporting both men who had tachycardia and were having breathing issues from the poisonous gases released from the exploding tank. We then helped to evacuate anyone in the immediate area and the rest of our shift was spent helping look after all of the firefighters on scene and supporting our fire family. I was wishing I was with them but that night I was well utilized and made the best of the bad situation despite almost having died. It wasn't until several years later when I looked at the actual pictures of the explosion at the fire school that I realized how lucky I truly was. The picture shows the explosion and the flying debris, which is bricks and sections of wall—all while I was crouching right next to the building. I don't know how or why I was spared that day but I'm so glad that day wasn't my last. It sure could have been if I was any slower or faster in any way.

One of my best days volunteering was when I responded a farm fire. We drove through the front gate and noticed the whole yard was on fire. All the outbuildings were starting to be affected and we attacked the fire. There was fire everywhere. I had never seen so much fire at one time. The poor family was about to lose everything. We fought that fire for hours and we had water tankers bringing us more and more water. We just kept spraying water and attacking one fire after another. After several hours, I was just exhausted. I was so hot and dry that I drank the water I was spraying and it never even mattered as it was already evaporated when it hit my lips, I'm sure. It was a team effort and we fought as one and we left as one even if we were physically depleted.

We took turns on the nozzle and then we would switch and pull or drag lines to the right place. When we got back to the hall that night it took us some time to get our trucks in order. Then we all sat around and shared our stories and I was shocked at what I had missed. I had been so involved in my own efforts that I hadn't noticed the huge effort of everyone else. That isn't my fault; it just shows you how important the other members of your crew are to you. You can't and will not see the effort of the big picture on the attack. The fire chief, the deputy chief and your fire captains are the ones saving your back. You might not see the hazards that can harm you as your field of vision is always too narrow.

This is very important to understand and I know several times in my life, my colleagues have saved me from harm when I missed the warning hazards. One time a car just missed me on the Wetaskiwin overpass at a MVC, but my firefighter friend grabbed me and pushed me out of the way. Another time I was at a MVC way out past Viking, when Mike Bye, an RCMP officer, moved me quickly when I wasn't watching my back and made sure I didn't get hit. For that and the many other times I've come close, I'm so thankful to my coworkers. I know I have helped many but many times in my life it was my coworkers who saved my life, as well.

*Chapter 18: University of Alberta Hospital – Stollery*

# "Making It Right"

I had the chance to work at the University of Alberta Hospital – Stollery (U of A) site from July 2002 for almost ten years. The experience was amazing, rewarding and something I will never forget. I went with the intention of learning and improving my skills and I got my money's worth and so much more. It was my internship to real critical care, and the only way to get the best education was to work with the best in the world. I was privileged and honoured to meet some of the best medical / surgical / critical care specialists in in the world.

The acuity was extremely high, as the level of care was at the highest in Alberta. But more important, I would learn to love my colleagues as my friends, then work beside them on the worst cases imaginable and help lead them on some of the worst shifts. These would be some of the best nurses, LPNs, respiratory therapists and support staff that I'd ever meet. Many are also the most dedicated and loyal friends I could ever ask for.

To this day, I will never forget the shifts from hell when we didn't think we would make it through the night. We worked as hard as humanly possible many times without breaks or a rest. We would work as quickly and as efficiently as possible to stabilize, then treat and transfer out or admit the patients who could have easily died without everyone's interventions. My memories of that time are, overall, some of the best of my career but, sadly, I ended up leaving due to my feelings of not being supported by management or feeling that I was actually needed. My colleagues and the staff I worked with were amazing but at the end of the day it was not enough when I was so worried about being set up to fail. I just felt like I was a number there, and that wasn't what I needed in life or would settle for, as life is too short. I needed to be supported and to know my back was covered as it was a high-stakes gamble saving lives and I was not going to be left without support.

But, as one door opens in life another must close. I will share some of the personal experiences and some very interesting lessons that come across my path on one of my many night shifts. A line from the movie, *Unconditional Joe*, sums it up my career at the University of Alberta Hospital – Stollery, all too well: "Life isn't a dead end if it takes you somewhere you needed to go." I got my fill of helping others at an all new level then I walked away before I could turn into a negative and not-as-effective leader.

During orientation, I was impressed at the flow of the patients and the unique way the hospital had of tracking patients, reviewing labs and assigning beds on the computer. It was amazing how after the triage process, a patient's file magically appeared in the complex system. The porters were on the ball, as well. Porters were always grabbing patients and helping them get to X-ray and back again in no time. Or, after we had a bed ready, we'd make a verbal report and a porter would assist a patient to a real bed.

Once a doctor assigned themselves to a patient, they were then responsible for the patient until disposition or admission. The doctors worked very hard to make sure patients had the best assessments, the complete diagnostic assessment or a complete lab assessment. Sometimes this was a little excessive but it was the trend at the time. Patients would not be able to get into a family doctor soon enough and would sometimes wait for months to see a specialist, but the ER was always open. You could get a complete assessment at no cost to you other than your time, and it was almost always worth it.

Sometimes the patients would be seen right away and then sent out the door in record time. And other times they were admitted and then got stuck in the emergency room (ER) for two to three days if there were no beds upstairs. This caused the bottlenecking of the system, which sucked for everyone, especially the patient in many cases. Although sometimes when they got up to some wards, looking back they maybe got better care in the ER depending on the variables. The system wasn't built by people who were staff nurses or had worked in the current present system.

Many hospitals or medically oriented building ideas or plans are based on presentation or looks and not on practicality. The developers would cut costs in places that were not logical, but common sense or practical reasons are not a high priority in many health care facilities. A hospital needs a better way of helping patients flow through the system more efficiently to be efficient and more practical. Sometimes we work on a wellness model and sometimes it's a sickness world model. Sometimes the combination of the two is tried, and fails or is a success depending on the people involved and the unique circumstances. No two patients or circumstances are ever the same. We need diversity and flexibility to be efficient.

The orientation process was a good long week and I was looking forward to the buddy shifts. Funny, they told me it would be about six months before I got to work in A-Pod which was the highest acuity pod and the place where the sickest patients were looked after. They also had a rule that you could not work in the busy University of Alberta Hospital – Stollery ER unless you had many years of experience but the new grads being hired displayed that wasn't the case anymore. In just over a week I would see the real ER in A-Pod. In just a week I was in A-Pod doing what I could there with my buddy, and it was just like a normal day. Saving lives and making it a better day for someone. My formal orientation was over and the real training was underway.

We had to run fast, think faster and have as much fun as possible to keep us from going insane. Compassion fatigue wasn't even considered. You never complained; you just went hard and kept up with the team. On your day off, you recharged, and when you walked out of the break room it was time for battle every time. Breaks were not mandatory but appreciated when you got them. I used mine to sleep, if possible, as the 3 to 4 hour drive per day and the twelve-hour shifts kept me maxed out. A few times I had to have a nap in the parkade after I had driven the ninety to one hundred-minute drive to work. It was worth the experience and the expert learning capabilities.

I will never forget the people I met and became friends with over the years while serving at the University of Alberta Hospital – Stollery ER. Early on, I befriended Marliese Pasay and didn't know then that she would become one of my very best friends. She eventually married Dr. Eddie Chang, one of the best critical care doctors I have ever met. Eddie had started as volunteer and worked his way to the top. I was more than lucky to work alongside Dr. Chan. Eddie also volunteered to be a medical director for some of the courses we taught all over Alberta. I knew Marliese had a good man to be her soul mate and it made me smile from ear to ear the day they got married. Robyn and I were privileged to witness the breathtaking ceremony of such a great couple.

The humblest and most sincere man I ever worked with was Ray Atkinson: a pure gentle giant and one of the most nonjudgmental people I ever met. He was at the U of A for as long as I can remember. In 1989 when we dropped off patients, he would have helped with our trauma orthopedic patients. Ray was an LPN / Ortho Tech and saved the ER physician time and time again by performing orthopedic-related cast and splint applications. Then years later,

I found out I would be working with him in ER at the U of A – Emergency Room.

Over the years I got to see the other side of Ray, which is the real Ray. Then he was promoted to my friend. He also became my golden retriever's best friend. Tinsel and Pebbles would always flank him when he comes to visit or babysit for my dogs. They were a match in heaven. They helped each other. Ray gives them unconditional love and they just adore him.

Ray and I have done many road trips together and for the last two years we toured the east coast and stayed with my friend, Troy Harnish, for a holiday of a lifetime. Troy was one of my friends that I would keep running into at work. On our first trip to the east coast I finally got to meet his partner, Bonnie. Then last year Ray and I were honoured to be guests at their wedding. Bonnie was raised in Newfoundland and the only way I could describe her is the salt of the earth. She is so infectious and caring, and never has a bad word to say about anybody. So, working at the U of A kept me seeing other friends from other parts of my life which was very fulfilling. It was not uncommon for me to meet many past students while on shift in the ER as well.

The next person from those day whom I am privileged to call a friend is Dr. Kevin Nelson. I met Kevin as a STARS physician back when I was a STARS nurse and I never forgot him. More important, I got to know him outside of the hospital and went to his place many times where I got to see how dedicated he is to his wife Karen, whom I also worked with at the University of Alberta. I also got to meet his rescue family, which consisted of some amazing dogs, so like my own. You could not find a gentler soul on the planet: a very strong methodical man who was so full of wisdom in many areas and not just medicine. I got to know and trust him when I was having so much trouble in my life. I could always talk to him and we would come up with a solution. But the most remarkable time was one dark night that I will never forget. You wont know who is your friend until you call them and as a mere miracle they answer on the third ring.

One evening, my kids, Evan and Robyn, and I had gone over to visit my friends, Ray and Darlene, in Edmonton to help move some gravel and yard bricks. They were two of my good friends from the University of Alberta and they need some help and we volunteered. I was taking our van but in the last second, I decided to take my F-250 Diesel 4x4 extended cab truck to help just in case we needed to haul stuff for them. We got the job done in no time; we had a quick coffee then headed home as it was getting dark. We turned off Highway 14 onto Highway 21 and Evan was driving. I told him to be extra careful and watch out for moose as this was their home territory. I didn't want to hit a moose as that would be bad for all of us. We had gone about ten miles and we had a little car right on our bumper. We had just passed a car, and right there coming straight at us was the moose I warned Evan about. He turned slightly left toward the centre lane to try to miss it but it was too late. We took Mr. Moose out with extreme prejudice. Most of the damage was on the right front of the truck. Thankfully, we hit him instead of the car with three people in it that was going to pass us. They would have all died. Our lights went out and the engine died right then. Evan somehow managed to pull the truck over to the right side in the blackness. We were alive and that was all that mattered. It could have been much worse.

While we were stopped, and sitting there, we tried to find our phones but there was almost no light. The car behind us stopped without hitting us or the moose. We had a quick look and the moose was dead. I finally found our phone and called 911. I then called Kevin, who lived closer than anyone else I knew, and he answered right away. In less than ten minutes, he was there along with the closest RCMP and made our day better and rescued us all.

Kevin gathered up the kids and their stuff into his truck to be safe. We were out on the busy highway with no lights and our truck was dark, lifeless and dead, so it was still not exactly safe. We grabbed our personal effects and then we looked at my truck. The moose took the whole right-hand front side off and destroyed it and then it hit my passenger side window so hard with its head, I suspect, that it dented inward. We were sprayed with glass and now the whole front seat was littered with glass and we only had a few small scratches to show for it. Miracles do happen and this was one of them.

Kevin took us to Camrose, following the tow truck, and retrieved the remainder of my personal stuff as it was never going to be my truck again. Then he got us home that night and would not even consider any payment. That is who Kevin was. Someone you could count on 24/7. I also got to see the real Kevin on night shifts and he was one person who I could always rely on when I needed help or backup in any event. Even today I know I can call him any time of the day or night and he would be at my side no matter the reason.

The other part of my U of A experience consisted of the patients that we triaged, assessed and worked on daily. The most patients we ever had in the waiting room at any one time was about fifty, but it was not uncommon to have fifteen to twenty always waiting to be seen. We had anywhere from forty-five to fifty beds that were constantly being filled and emptied. On my worst night about thirty of these beds were filled with admitted patients and we had eighteen ambulances waiting. I worked extra hard as the charge nurse to get people in and out, but sometimes you can't win the battle. We never got the waiting room emptied by the end of my shift and as the sun started to come up, people started coming to fill up the waiting room all over again. The cycle was never the same from day to night and some days it never stopped or slowed down. What made it work was the amazing nurses, doctors, porters, radiology staff, respiratory therapists and clerks who made the system function. One of the basic survival skills you needed to know was who you could count on in each pod. That way when all hell hit the fan you always had backup and you used them often.

One thing I really liked about working at the U of A was the multicultural aspect. People came from all over the world and we were working together in one building for one reason: to help people no matter who they were or why they were there. They would all get treated the same. It was not somewhere that religion or colour mattered and that was something I really appreciated. I had seen many places where it was not this good. I had been in other places, such as Wetaskiwin, where prejudice had harmed and even killed. I had a child die on me because a physician was a racist. I said never again. If it meant losing my licence, then so be it. Not on my watch. I don't care what race or colour you are or what religious beliefs you may have or what level of education you've attained; if you're sick, I will help you.

One of the nights I will never forget was the night I was supposed to be the charge nurse and it was one of my first shifts where I was trying to make it all function without letting the walls fall. Just after I started, a lady came running in carrying a younger child. I could tell right away something was wrong. I ran to meet her. I took one look at this little guy and I could see we were in trouble. The child was in full cardiac arrest. I grabbed him and ran back to a resuscitation room, yelling as I went through the doors of pediatric ward "Code Blue!" Everyone on the ward came to my rescue right away. I remember the pediatrician at my side working frantically to get the little child going breathing again and everything we tried was in vain.

Nothing would help as we were too late in getting him. We coded the child for a long time and never got anything back. We had no significant history other than his not being well for a few days. No real sickness or any signs of trauma. Sadly, he died from something very rare in children: he had a gastrointestinal bleed for some strange reason. I would have not believed it f I wasn't there, but that was the final diagnosis. This is common in older patients or those with significant internal injuries but very rare in a happy kid with such a loving mother who has just lost everything valuable in her world.

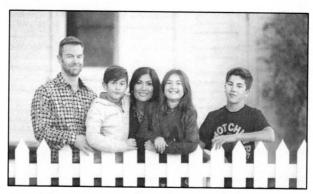

*Dr. Tim Graham, U of A ER / Staff Physician (a very proud dad and husband) and Dr. Samina Ali, U of A ER Pediatrician (a very brilliant, gifted doctor and such a gift to the pediatric world.) This remarkable lady showed me that I mattered. Samina also taught me to be a better person and even more forgiving of others in need of love and caring. I was so fortunate to work alongside both of these wonderful physicians on many long nights. Tim and Samina, your children are amazing—you are both so blessed. I will always be your loyal friend.*

Sometimes the shifts were bad but that night sucked the worst. The only good thing that night was that the staff stuck together and after the death was called, we had our moment together and we grieved as one. We hugged each other and shared some tears and we went on with the night. That was what we had to do.

Another one of my most memorable shifts started like so many others. The unrelenting waiting room kept filling up, there were more ambulances lined up than you could ever deal with and then the charge nurse's phone rang one more time. The call was a deployment. Seven kids had all been ejected at high speed and we were getting them all as they were all less than seventeen years old. All we knew was that the car had been travelling at a very high speed and two to three were critical. The rest were all red patients, which is bad as well. The only good news was that no one was dead. "Yet," I thought. "Not yet."

I walked quickly to the A-Pod to place a call to locate services. I asked them to notify the trauma team, the OR staff, the pediatric on-call ICU staff, all surgical residents and on-call staff that they could roundup. We even got anesthesiology ready and waiting just in case, as pediatric airway disasters are unforgiving even with the best ER doctors in the world. The respiratory therapist found us more RTs and we were as ready as we could be in no time. I also got permission to re-route any incoming ambulances to other hospitals if possible.

We needed at least three trauma teams and we needed them in less than ten minutes. When I got to A-Pod, we had a quick huddle and made a working plan. We completely emptied out A-pod and got three stations besides our trauma X-ray room ready to rumble. We would meet this disaster head on and we would save as many as we could. Just as the first kids arrived so did a walk-in with s stab or gunshot wound to the chest. I can't for the life of me remember which it was but we took him as well and never even batted an eye.

The staff that night was fantastic. Other than the fact that I was making the other pods angry with me as I pulled a few staff from each one to help with the disaster. We had one very experienced critical care doctor or PICU staff and one surgical staff at each patient and we attacked. In no time, we had them stabilized and slowly started getting porters to take them to the waiting pediatric operating room (OR) or to the PICU, as most appropriate. We saved them all and we made it through the night even without any other complications. That would be one of most successful nights I had in my career, knowing I was the leader and we went to war with the worst-of-the-worst trauma and we won. That morning I drove home and don't even know how I made the 100-km drive in one hour and forty-five minutes as I was so dead tired. After working twelve hours straight plus driving 100 km each way, I had reached my breaking point. I needed a few hours' sleep and in six hours I had to be ready to do it all over again. We, the caretakers and the evil, the heartbreakers, had battled one more time. This time we won and the grim reaper lost.

As one of a few male nurses in the department, I was often called when my coworkers needed help and several times when they or someone else was being attacked, either physically or verbally. We took on the role with no question, and a few times I even got hurt in the process but it was worth the stitches every time. Nurses like Big John whose voice could wake the dead, Greg Siefert, Gary Lundman and Dave Trabish were people who could always be counted on n the times of need. We never hurt anyone but we got control of the situation, performed many surgical takedowns in the interest of protecting the public, and ultimately saved our patients and coworkers from a worse fate.

We didn't have on a cape, but when called we were right there. We saved each other and many of our coworkers still today say thanks for saving them when they had no backup in sight. Nursing management, on the other hand, had told us to look the other way. I was told a woman could be in the middle of being punched and my role as a nurse was to look the other way and eventually security would come and deal with the problem. I think not. CARNA, our nursing body, investigated me for stopping a person after he punched a nurse in the face while his family just looked on and watched. They claimed I held him too firmly. This was so we could medicate him and take him to the CT scanner to ensure he didn't have an active cerebral or brain bleed, and was not just a class-A asshole. Not sure how or why some people think they can spit on us, punch us or even kick us and then claim they were not in their right minds so it didn't happen. As it turned out, his CT scan showed nothing abnormal so he was "in his right mind" at the time.

As a charge nurse, I wasn't always just walking around and harassing the staff to work harder or double-checking if they were doing their job—that wasn't my role. Our job was to make sure the patients got through the system without delay, with the most appropriate care, and that staff had the resources to do their job. Some patients were heavy in the amount of the workload they would require while others were super easy. One night I got a little too committed to my work and it turned out to be a night that I won't ever forget. We had survived a cold winter night without much going wrong until 5:00 a.m. Then all hell broke loose.

The patient had been stabbed in the chest and this meant it was either fatal right away, or the patient would lose pulse in a short time and we'd attempt an open thoracotomy, in which case almost all patients will die anyway. In my history, I have helped with five such cases, and two survived to walk out of hospital while three were just as dead as a turd in a milk bucket you might say. This night, the patient was hypotensive right away and was about 70/ systolic. EMS came right in with her and we took her to A-Pod. In no time, we were losing her. She had a huge cardiac silhouette that was larger than it should have been. One of the stab wounds had most likely punctured the pericardium, which is the thin double-walled fibrous sac surrounding the heart. The blood would leak out of the stab wound and then it would be stuck sitting in this space and, slowly, the space the heart needs to beat disappears. Cardiac arrest is inevitable in these cases. All you can do is preload the heart and get a thoracic surgeon or someone very skilled to perform a thoracotomy immediately or they will die.

We were fortunate that night as the staff physician had performed these procedures multiple times and the surgeon on call just happened to come in at the right time. Our emergency physician was intubating and pushed the endotracheal tube in deeper than normal for the surgeon to cut the chest wall open on the left side to have direct access to the heart. As soon as he started cutting, I realized he didn't even have time to apply the scalpel to a handle. He was cutting as fast as humanly possible with the blade firmly grasped between his fingers. Once he got into the space around the heart after cutting the pericardial sac open, he could see the damage. But the heart lacked the appearance of normal as it was empty and not pumping. It looked to be completely collapsed with no volume left. We could not suction fast enough so I took the Yankauer suction tip off and suctioned with straight suction tubing, with the surgeon suctioning and then sticking his fingers in the hole in the heart.

It was funny timing, as my charge phone started to ring and someone had to fish it out of my pocket as I was slightly committed to being a scrub nurse for a few minutes. The holes were sutured and the heart had to be shocked with little internal probes a few times, all while the IVs and blood were being run wide open. In no time, the heart took form and suddenly it was pumping and we had a pulse. This is one time BP is sort of optional: if you can see the heart working and give it something to pump, it will work. Take away the cardiac tamponade and the tension pneumothorax and it wants to pump all on its own.

The funniest and scariest cardiac tamponade I helped save was strange as I didn't see it coming until it was too late. My patient was having a rough night. His friend had stabbed him not because of hate or anything—just too much alcohol and a sharp knife being at the wrong place at the wrong time. Our CT scanner was broken so I had to take him up straight to diagnostic imaging (DI) and as soon as I took one look at the CT scout while the CT tech was getting the patient ready, I almost yelled out "Shit!" as the patient had a huge bulging of the pericardial sac in the left upper side of his heart visible on the CT scout. We completed the scan quickly and I rolled him back to the ER as fast as possible. I knew if he arrested in the hallway or elevator we were doomed. At least back in the ER I had friends who could deal with this crisis quickly. Surgical intervention was the only option and at any time he could go into cardiac arrest. "Not on my shift," I was praying.

I called the cardiovascular (CV) resident he was on his way and, luckily, Harvey the senior surgical resident happened to walk into the trauma X-ray room known as A-6 right after I called for help stat. Harvey was an amazing and gifted surgical resident. I'd known him for some time and was happy to see him. Shortly after, I had the patient back on the monitor and the vitals were stable. The oxygen probe was showing me a great wave form and the numbers were good, so I thought we were golden. We were getting ready for disaster but I wasn't the bus driver of fate that night. But I sure as heck made the right decision in calling for help right away.

The CV resident had arrived as well, assessed him and was calling the OR when it all went sideways. I looked up to see the SpO2 wave-forms just die off. I knew this was because the cardiac tamponade had caused the patient to go into cardiac arrest. This is thought to happen as the amount of the fluid had gone past the magic cusp that had pushed the patient into a state of not being able to pump anymore. If you could drain off 10 to 20 mLs, the heart might have had room to pump but we didn't have any time to do that. Also, the heart was leaking so fast it was a waste of time anyway. The leak was bigger than you could compensate for. When someone drives a big knife into your heart and pulls it out, the damage is done.

I yelled at the CV surgeon for help. He told me they could have an OR in an hour, and I said we need one in five minutes as he's dead in ten. Harvey knew what to do and in a flash, he had a scalpel in his hand and was cutting the chest open. In no time, he had the pericardial sac visible. When he cut the pericardial sac, the blood went everywhere. It was a bloodbath all over that side of the room and over the IV cart. He immediately stuck his finger in the hole directly into the heart itself. I looked up and the SpO2 waveform was coming back almost immediately. The miracles of a thoracotomy when done by the right person, at the right time, with the patient in just the right place are astonishing.

Almost immediately the patient came back from his near-death experience. I bet you can't get any closer to the light than that and come back without CPR or any medications being administered. His eyes opened wide and he let out a moan. I'm sure having your chest cut wide open even while shock was very painful. I still can see his eyes opening bigger and bigger by the second. You didn't need a BP to know he was back alive. Death had been aborted at least for a while, and as long as Harvey plugged the hole and we filled his gas tank up quickly with IV fluid and blood products, he'd likely live to show off a nasty chest scar. We medicated him right away and intubated him at the same time. In a short period, they had an OR ready. This poor man needed some amazing surgical expertise.

I still remember the green towel draped over his heart that was lifting up and down with every heartbeat. So, in no time at all I had been in on and helped with two patients who had an open thoracotomy. It was a miracle; we had saved two separate stabbing patients who should have died. With the right people and the right team surgical miracles are performed. This is still one of my memorable saves that I was a part of. I just watched Harvey take over the job of the CV surgeon, who was holding on to the phone in shock I would think for most of the intervention. The final score was ER: 1 and the Grim Reaper: 0 that night.

After ten years, I'd had come to a roadblock in my career. My nights were always interesting and I always came across situations or events I had not seen or dealt with but we found a solution. Several times I was told I was catering too much to the EMS staff or to STARS instead of the waiting room patients and I ignored that comment. I went to Lesley, one of the most senior supervisors, when I felt I needed help. I admired her leadership and I always knew she had my back, as I had worked many hellish shifts right beside her.

I actually would have taken a bullet or a knife or done anything for her. I would have died for her. I just wanted her to be my boss or my clinical staff to be in my corner. I told her I wanted someone I trusted with my life. I wanted someone I knew that was on my side if I was right and if I was wrong then I was wrong. If I was wrong Lesley would have told me, and I would have accepted it on the spot. I would admit to her when I was wrong because I knew she would know why I went out of my way to save lives or help people. Lesley knew me for years and she trusted me to make the right decision when it counted.

If a management team or a management style fails, then the whole system fails. I didn't want to be just a number anymore. Plus, the driving was killing me and after working hard for twelve hours and trying to drive 200 km a day in all kinds of road conditions I could not keep doing it safely. I was going to a place I didn't want to be. It was affecting my life and if I kept going, something bad would happen. Twice I had fallen asleep driving home after a night shift. I could not kill myself or worse yet kill someone else because I wasn't getting enough sleep. I had to think of a better work plan before fate made my plan for me.

Then after the night my dad died I took of a few shifts off for the funeral. I knew after that that I was nothing to them as not one person called me or even asked me how I was doing. Many of the staff on the floor had shown support but when it came to management I got zero. My fellow EMS staff had called me multiple times and was checking up on me faithfully. I knew they mattered to me and I mattered to them. I just didn't understand why my nursing managers didn't care. I worked very hard, but for what cost I started to think? When doubt creeps in to your mind you're already beat. That hurt me greatly, knowing on many nights I'd stuck my neck out to help others but, apparently, it wasn't enough. I thought they were my family too but I guess I was wrong and that was that. If I'm wrong, then I'm wrong. If I was just filling a spot on the schedule and that was it, I wasn't the right person anymore.

So, after another bad night of way too many ambulances waiting to offload, and way too many patients waiting to be admitted to the ER with no more beds to assess patients, I was broken. I had seen a patient die because he had to wait in the waiting room for about seven hours with a dissecting aneurysm. In the end, he might have died anyway but at least we could have helped alleviate some of the pain. He died a long painful death, mostly in the waiting room, with management in their office pushing more papers but not helping us fix the real problem. The system let everyone down that day. We all failed the patient; we failed the family. I had only come onto my shift long enough to help get him after they transported him off the waiting room floor. I started my shift in C-Pod with a buddy nurse.

I was called to help and my buddy took over my patients. The man was put on the first available ER stretcher and sent off to an A-Pod bed, then off to the CT scanner for the already bad news. Then from there it was managing his pain and dealing with his angry family. The OR was not an option due to the already severe internal damage and he would not survive the OR table anyway. By midnight, it was over, and it was one of the worst shifts I can remember. It will always be about eleven hours of the worst pain and suffering I had seen that I'm sure will haunt that poor family for ever. It was not my fault. It was not my coworkers' fault. It was the system's fault and nothing can fix a broken system but pushing for change to prevent similar episodes.

The thing I will never forget was one of the relatives was a senior police officer who had worked the streets for years. I was talking to him and I was also very upset the system had failed them at all levels. Then he told me something I had never thought about even after seeing the most violent deaths and the pure evil that society has to offer. He said it so right that night that we have saved many that could and should have died. I had seen the miracles of what we had done in the EMS world many times but never actually put the facts together. I had no clue we were changing destiny as a team.

I had witnessed and seen the problems from an outside perspective many times so he knew it wasn't always our fault when things went wrong. The system had its faults and you couldn't always win. One scary example he told me that I never even considered was that street violence in the city was getting worse but we were getting better at saving the people who should be dead. We had learned the deadly dozen and also shared the wisdom with the EMS and rural hospital over and over.

The EMS was so good at grabbing the critical patients from the scenes and heading immediately to one of the two local trauma hospitals. They aborted death and even patients in cardiac arrest were brought back and saved by the gifted medical and surgical staff. Someone had the intention to kill someone else and we ruined their plans from time to time. Occasionally these patients actually walked into the ER or a loving family member dropped them off at the front door. I've seen some walk in and then die in a very short time despite our best efforts.

I have even been on one of these teams and made mistakes myself and thankfully none of them have been fatal. One time this happened as a person walked out of our hospital and then stabbed himself many times. He was immediately brought back in and we did our best to keep him alive despite the fact that he wanted to die very badly. Just the day before the vials of morphine were changed from one colour to another as well as the concentrations were also reversed. This creates medication mistakes in times of a crisis. Dr. Rowe was in charge of the trauma team. I was pushing drugs to help intubate the patient. I grabbed the syringe and someone had loaded it with the morphine. I could see green on the tape and Dr. Rowe yelled out the drug he wanted. I grabbed it and pushed the plunger and I was giving even less than he called for but unbeknownst to me I just gave 10 mg instead of the 2 mg I thought I had given.

As soon as I realized it, I admitted it to everyone in the room. Then Dr. Rowe looked at me and yelled, "Are you trying to kill my patient?" I was embarrassed but I also knew the patient had done his best with a knife to kill himself already. Also, people missed the part that he was a patient of ours and was just discharged and the whole time he had the knife and could have hurt anyone of us. Twice now I have seen patients leave the ER and kill the taxi driver or someone who least was expecting it. You're never as safe as you think with people who are mentally ill or in a drug-induced psychosis. We need to always watch each other's backs and know that any time your life can be challenged with lethal force.

Thankfully, the amount I gave still wasn't enough to kill him and we had to give him more than expected. I learned an important lesson; I was the teacher of this lesson for years before and I just got caught making the same mistake. I knew better. But for years the green vials were 2 mg and one day the system changed the dosages. They say about 50 per cent of drug errors are actually system errors. I always have and will keep my guard up for concentration errors and medication dosages as I have been caught and have seen my coworkers and others make these same mistakes.

We meet all kinds of people and some of our patients are not very nice to us at times. Some people would come in and ask for help but in the end, they actually walked out with severe injuries before we were able to help them. When someone has the ability to harm us or refuses care, their ultimate destiny rests on their shoulders and not ours.

As a charge nurse, it was a constant fight with other wards to take patients to make more room for the ones waiting to come in. One Friday night a ward would not take our patient as they declared it would be unsafe. The patient was over at Timmy's on his own and in no acute distress. He was only being admitted to get an MRI on Monday and then could be seen by the specialist. It doesn't get any easier to babysit a patient who isn't even in the building. But when you're that lazy and your coworkers allow it or even promote this behaviour it becomes toxic.

One Sunday night I'd had enough and wrote my resignation letter and walked away knowing the system would just keep getting worse and slowly the new nurses would be required to take over even if they were headed to a pending disaster. I resigned and walked away from ten of the best years of my life. I just can't go down a road that I don't want to walk down if in my heart, I know it isn't right. Life is way too short not to have job satisfaction. You can't care for others properly when you're not being cared for by your own people.

To the winners in life, you will always need to draw your line in the sand and make your stand on your own terms. Never give into what you know is wrong and not right despite the modified society rules. You must follow your personal code or standards that guide your ethics to do what is right. Sometimes you have to make your stand regardless of the people against you, then you must declare your beliefs and make them known to the ones involved. That is what makes winners win. Winners save lives. Winners make the right decisions for the right reasons.

The coolest part about being one of the dedicated, hardworking charge nurses was that you got the trust of so many people. The staff got to know you and would back you up or help you in a heartbeat. An example was when I called one of our very busy ER physicians and asked for treatment options, he was very frank with me. He said, "Dale, do whatever the hell you want, but don't make me lose my licence," and hung up on me and got back to saving a life. That right there is trust that is earned. Another time I called one of our senior doctors for help. He said he'd come right away because of one word. I simply told him our patient, whom we were trying to stabilize, had stopped breathing again. He said it was the "again" part that hit it home to him that this was something a little more serious than his other concerns right now. That made me smile from ear to ear.

Even after I quit, I still got to see many of the friends I'd made at the U of A over the years. Many of them wanted me to be their teacher for any ACLS or PALS courses they had to take every two years. I even taught courses at some of their houses as a big group where we'd have so much fun it was hard to believe that it was a course about life and death. By teaching my friends, we raised over $50,000.00 to help the Alberta Heart and Stroke Association. After about two or three years we decided to also support other causes. We then took the money we raised from the courses and gave it to the Stollery Pediatric Neurosurgery Fund after we made our original goal of $50,000.00.

So at the end of the day, it's a really small word and almost everything we do feeds the circle of life in some form or fashion. Not a day goes past that I don't miss the people from the University of Alberta Hospital - Stollery but it was time for change. Change brings growth and growth brings wisdom. Often, I would call my friend Kevin and ask him how he was doing and he would always reply with, "Don't know." Kevin, who is one of the best ER doctors I've worked with, would usually say to me next, "I know nothing and I can prove it." Well, I can tell you I know even less. I can prove that when I measure myself against most of my friends. They are the people that matter. They are the people who save lives day in and day out.

Dale M. Bayliss

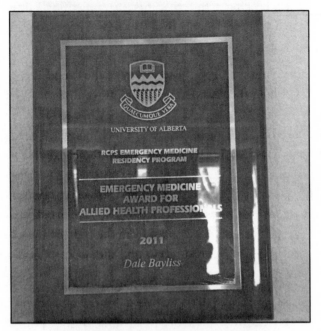

*"It was an amazing and challenging part of
my life. The rewards were lifelong."*

# "Saving Lives 101"

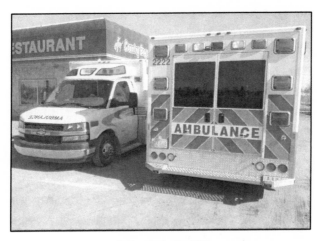

*"The Right Stuff"*

I have been working for Beaver EMS for over ten years now. We respond as a solo crew or as two crews and we always have each other's backs and that is appreciated. No matter what call comes in, I always try to get to the scene first even if it means speeding just a bit. I have been pulled into the office a few times to be reminded of response rules and I listen carefully and then go back to work. It is part of management's role to ensure we follow the rules that are dictated by the upper crust in our provincial EMS management. Some have little awareness of the rural requirements or ignore them and only address the urban concerns. But we make it work no matter the limitations or the scrutiny we are under 24/7. Somehow the rural and urban EMS are still not seen as equals by some people in power.

243

Several times the city supervisors actually told me the rural areas didn't matter and the urban people did so I would just do what I was told and they would help free up only the urban crews. They had no idea how dumb or silly they sounded but we always did our best to get the hell out of the city and get back to our rural communities, despite the unfair treatment by a few people in power. I signed up to help my people in Beaver County for a reason and my reason was simple and easy to understand. They mattered just as much as anyone else. People everywhere mattered to me and I would show that over and over again in my career. I loved the staff at the local rural hospitals as well and they always made me feel welcome. Tofield and Viking staff were what made helping people the best part. They cared and they never ever parked us in the hallways just because they could. That actually saved a few lives, I'm positive.

We have the right people and the right equipment to make the difference in many lives. We have many people working for us who are the best of the best. We have amazing crew members who have dedicated their lives to helping others. Not all staff we've had have been rock stars but on average they are better than most. Another reason I wanted to work at Beaver EMS was that I knew we were a team. When we go to calls, it is as one.

Several times I made the first on-call crew mad as we were the second crew out and we could still beat them to the scene. I said to one of paramedics after he complained to actually "Give a shit" and make the call the priority and not take the allowable seven minutes to get out the door. Then you can always be first to the scene. He shut up and we took the patient that he never really wanted to look after, anyway. It was the only service I worked for that had the best equipment, the best staff and we didn't have to fight to get paid. Our sleeping quarters were private and the showers, the bays and units were clean, so it was a win-win.

The best thing about Beaver EMS is that the equipment we have has always been good. We had the best cardiac monitors even before the other services had the LP 12s and we were one of the first to get the new video laryngoscopes on every unit. Our front-line units all have the Lucas CPR devices and it makes doing a cardiac arrest on patients so much better when they fit. If the patient is over 100 pounds or less than 300 pounds they will fit the machine, and it makes chest compressions much more effective in most situations. Many years ago, we also had the Genesis Ventilators that were a unique device for proving artificial ventilations when they were used but not appropriate in all cases. Looking back, Beaver EMS has been a very progressive and dedicated ALS service that has a reputation for saving lives despite the expected tragic outcomes. We make a difference in thousands of lives over the years.

One of the cases I will never forget at Beaver EMS was a call that makes you wonder what I can do next to change the best results and come out of a bad situation. I don't always know what is best but sometimes you only have a few options and you do what you can. We were called to a patient having a seizure in a rural location. This is a common call but, in no time, this call would be the most complicated and complex seizure call I had ever seen and it would test us all. On scene, we arrived to find a complex scene and a much more complex call. We had a patient having a grand-mal seizure on the second level of a big metal Quonset. But the problems were much more complex. He was up about sixteen feet from the ground and the only way to get him out was by a spiral staircase. So, extrication was going to be a bigger problem. We had to stop the seizure first, then stabilize him and also find a way to get him down to our unit. But the first question was why did he have the seizure? This was my only question that needed an immediate answer. In no time, I had the answer, even if I couldn't prove it.

After I took my first real look at look at him I knew right away he was in big trouble. He looked to be pale as a ghost. I assessed him and we got him supine right away. The oxygen was applied with a face mask and an IV was started and was now running wide open with just normal saline. I actually knew the patient but not well as he had some medical history from the past that was very significant. About six months ago, I had him as a patient on a routine transfer and I knew he had some strange internal bleeding disorder. I had spent time reading his past medical history on the transfer sheet and it made me wonder even then what would cause the bleeding concerns.

Now, he was unresponsive and having a seizure on our arrival so any extra history I wanted from him wasn't an option at all. I was just thinking and I came up with a differential diagnosis and I knew we would treat him for that. If I was wrong I was wrong but if I was right we would save a life. We needed to at least head that direction and if it was meant to be we would win.

I called for them to dispatch the local fire department and requested we launch STARS and I asked for a favour. "Bring me blood," I said. Then I added, "Lots of it." The fire crews were on scene right away and were asked to set up a landing spot just outside the building. They also had to help with the extrication so they would be extra busy tonight. But today the plan was changed in a hurry. STARS had the blood and were willing to come but the bad weather prevented a launch. We were having a bad storm and it was coming right at us.

I had to come up with a Plan B and it was already on my mind. I called the critical care line and they linked us to the STARS physician, as well as the Viking physician. Dr. Cunningham knew us all too well even if he always called me Kevin, but that was a compliment in my eyes. I said I needed the blood on scene for our patient. In a second Dr. Cunningham had it ready by getting the lab tech to grab it and it was ours for the getting. I called in another favour and in minutes, blood was coming to us. I had the Rural Regional Fire Chief coming to Viking Hospital to get it in minutes. We got the right approval from the right people and the blood was coming to me in the fire chief's truck, lights-and-sirens. It's good to have friends in this world.

We would stabilize the patient and then extricate him with the fire department doing a rope rescue over the side wall and down the sixteen feet to our waiting stretcher. Then when the blood arrived it would be administered. Unbeknownst to me, we had a severe lightning and rain storm also coming right at us, which would make our transport even more challenging. We also had the RCMP on scene and they were my Plan C. In no time, we had fluid boluses in our patient and we were getting him more stable but he still needed the blood. It was a temporary fix but it was a start. It could wait for a bit as we had aborted the seizure and broken the complications down by getting his brain perfused with essential fluid and with oxygen. He was even waking up despite looking as if he needed about three or four units of blood as soon as possible. Any time you have a patient waking up, you're doing something right.

The Holden volunteer firefighters were amazing. We had the patient safety tied into a STOKES basket and lowered over the support wall and down the sixteen foot drop without incident. This was at the same time as providing oxygen and lifesaving IV therapy so it was not as easy as you might think. He was wheeled to the unit and we made another plan. The rain was just starting to hit us. The winds were just starting to shake our unit, as well. The RCMP were meeting us at the local Holden ESSO. As soon as we got to the meeting spot I had come up with an alternate plan, I had a good backup plan ready to go. I knew we would make it work. We had to. We were going to win this battle.

Plan C was to get the fire chief to drive until we would hit the city limits. I had commandeered a volunteer firefighter, Heather, to help me in the back to squeeze the bulb on the pressure infusers and help change the pressure infuser on the IV bags and then on the blood products as fast as possible. My partner Nathan was helping do everything else that I wasn't able to do or see. We had the perfect team. We had the blood tubing primed with normal saline in seconds and the lifesaving blood running wide open as soon as it could start dripping in was running. Nathan was doing vital signs and also making sure I wasn't missing anything. Nathan was an amazing partner. I knew that day he would rock as a paramedic in the future. We took off for the city, with the RCMP making the traffic split right down the middle, and were headed right for the storm. We were being pelted with rain and the high winds and we never looked back for it was the night for speed.

Following us, we had the fire rescue truck bringing up the rear and they would take our volunteer firefighters back as soon as we got to the city hospital. All this was being monitored by the dispatch centre and critical care was kept updated as well. We had the STARS physician on the line as well who was also listening to our conversations and helping us make important decisions. It was common for me to just place the call and then put my iPhone down and leave it on speaker so everyone could hear or talk when it was needed. We were one hell of a team and we were making it better by supporting each other. Our dispatcher that night was also amazing. There is always stuff happening behind the scenes that they were doing that we never even heard. They were getting us to the right hospital. They also had patched us into the right critical care physicians and were making sure everyone was aware of the progress as the night unfolded.

En route to the city hospital I asked if we could stop and grab some Pantoloc from the Tofield Health Centre as we passed it, as it would help decrease the bleeding, but the physician who was on-call that night was not so helpful. He actually told the STARS physician we were not allowed to stop and grab the medication which made no sense to me at all. All I wanted was the drug and he would never even see our patient but he was refusing anyway. The STARS doctor said, "Don't worry about it. It's not worth the hassle." So, we kept going at lightning speed, heading toward our critical care backup site. We were going as fast as possible and we had no problems with traffic as the cars got out of our way as we went past. It was not as fast as the STARS helicopter but we made really good time considering we were driving right through a storm.

On arrival at the city limits, I got Nathan to take over driving. When you're driving lights and siren in an ambulance, it is not as easy as it looks. I wanted to ensure we had no near misses in the city as we had some very important people to keep safe. All of us mattered and we would not take a chance on a crash. Our police escort also was in on our plans and they turned around and headed back home at the city limits. We were now dropping out of warp speed and we would have and efficient but safe drive for the rest of the trip.

On arrival, the staff where waiting for us and they rapidly took over our patient's care, and we knew that he was now in the hands of the best people to deal with the bleeding disorder. Thankfully, I was 100 per cent right and I had figured out the cause of the seizure right away and everything we did was to ensure he was going to live with the right amount of care provided. Everyone involved that night helped to save a life. I was just the person giving suggestions and ensuring we would save a life even when the plans kept changing. We never gave in to the roadblocks and we changed our plans to make it work the right way the first time.

The ride home that night was so uplifting. When we talked about what had happened and what could have happened, it was very satisfying. It showed me we have to always do our best for our patients at all times. If we just go to work and only give 70 per cent to 80 per cent effort on calls like this one, we would most likely have had a very different outcome. I had the right to give this patient multiple seizure medications, which would have made his condition worse and then I'd likely have had to intubate him. Then we would have had to fight with the severe hypotension that would follow our medication's side effects. Anything I tried would just increase the complications. So, by following protocol I could have actually caused more harm to the patient or even killed him. I might have easily been justified to follow the protocol and no one would have even faulted me. I went with what I knew in my heart and it was the best decision. Always assess and reassess your patient and listen to your partners and listen to your monitors, as well.

After many bad or complex calls, we would come back and our unit would be trashed. We would have blood on everything. All of our kits were torn apart. We had many calls like this and every time I came back to the base I could see the same style of leadership that showed Wes Baerg's true colours. Cheryl Cameron and Dan Schmick were the same and always made my team feel as if we counted as they never forgot about us as supervisors. Wes would be the first one out to help us tear the mess away from our unit and was right out there helping us to get our unit back in service, which was always our priority. We had another supervisor who would hide in the office and was no part of the team and that is why he didn't last.

Most of us always wanted to do the EMS calls as well as the transfers that come in at all hours. We had a community that counted on us 24/7. We always gave 110 per cent to everyone and never tried to get out of calls, not like other places I had seen in the past. Sadly, this happened one day when there was a cardiac arrest a few blocks away and the two closest crews argued over who should actually respond when it was clearly a crisis situation. Sadly, the outcome was terrible but nothing happened because no one cared about him. I knew the patient as he had worked with us, and the system might just have killed him. When you have a broken system with broken leadership the problem is never even addressed; it's just ignored. That day a man died and the system never even noticed until it was too late.

Another example was a crew that was always taking a forty-five-minute break after each call or transfer. They had a student in the car and the student called me and I could hardly believe it, but I had seen this behaviour in the past and the management looked the other way. That behaviour would kill me. They were not like me and never would be that dedicated. I'd fire them all in a heartbeat if I could but, thankfully, those crews were few in number or we would have been in big trouble on our busy days. Thank God, the majority of crews had brains, ambition and were dedicated to proving that patient care was needed to make a difference. When you care, it isn't work at all; it's a way of life. I go to work to have fun and fun I will have as long as I'm still alive.

Another great part about Beaver EMS was that they were always willing to support my "Give Back" programs. Even though we provided our time for free for the ACLS and PALS courses, we needed the extra equipment. Wes, along with Kevin, was more than helpful with this and allowed us to borrow the equipment we needed to provide the courses over the last five years in Viking and Tofield.

Wes also let us utilize the SUV and supported our PTSD walks over the last two years and that means so much. Crystal helped organize the BBQ after our walks and that was very important, as well. Many others around the world noticed our little effort to help others and slowly we got the message out. People from all over followed our walk on Facebook last year and we got so much encouragement. Last year alone we raised over $5000.00. This isn't much but it helps our Alberta Paramedic Association in times of crisis when an EMS member is killed or dies in the province. Money raised goes toward the surviving family and that is a great step to helping people that matter, at least in my book of life. I know it's not enough but it's a start, and that is the best I can offer some days.

The final case I want to share with you is one that proved when you expect the worst, every little thing you do can change the outcome to be a bit better. This particular call was sounding tragic right from the start. My partner and I thought it was going to be just another traumatic arrest and in a few minutes, it would be called and over. But that night we were wrong. That night we helped change destiny, even when we thought we were beaten before we started.

On our dispatch, we were told it was a car versus a pedestrian on the main highway. Seeing as it was dark and way past sundown, it wasn't hard to understand why someone could be hit walking down the highway at night. On this night, it was darker than usual and the moon and stars were hiding from sight. It would almost be impossible to see someone at night, especially if they had on dark clothes.

On arrival, we found the RCMP and the local fire department staff doing their best. Upon their arrival, they had found a patient in the ditch and thought she was already dead. They had poor lighting and did the right thing of taking her up to the road way to start CPR. If you think a patient is in cardiac arrest, you are 100 percent right to get them in a position to start CPR as spinal care doesn't really matter anymore. The damage is already done. When you get hit by a truck at highway speeds and thrown, if you're still alive it's a miracle. You were meant to live. But surprisingly to us she was still alive with poor breathing and the fire crew did their best to get her breathing right and applied oxygen and awaited our arrival.

As we walked up I was also shocked to see she was alive. Dave assessed her as well and in a second we had a plan. We needed to package her quickly and move her to the unit and get a proper airway right away. We knew for sure she had a traumatic head injury as well as her arm and leg were broken but if your still alive after all those injuries, with that significant mechanism of injury its nothing short of a miracle. It looked like the mirror on the truck had clipped her and the truck had most likely run over her foot and thrown her like a rag doll into the ditch. Once we got in the unit I did a good BP and confirmed in my mind her brain was most likely in trouble from the severe trauma. This is so common right after a severe head injury but I had a trick or two I learned from the people who were also my friends at the Advanced Trauma Life Support (ATLS) courses. Dr. Mary Stephens, Dr. Peter Bindley and Dr. Broad (the neurosurgeon) had made some very important points crystal clear on many occasions when it comes to supporting patients with severe head injuries.

It was very clear to me that night we needed to get the patient intubated upon arrival. Next, we needed to get the ventilations to the proper rate to keep the $CO_2$ at exactly 35 to save the brain. An important learning tip Dr. Peter Brindley had made sure everyone, including myself, understood was that the $CO_2$ waveform, when measured at the end of the endotracheal tube, was not calibrated the same as the blood gases. We were told to remember to always add plus three on our $CO_2$ monitor numbers to be more exact. So, we would need to over correct the $CO_2$ to someplace from 32 to 35 to save the brain. Just know if it says 40 you're at 43, approximately, is the best example about $CO_2$ levels. This won't matter in most cases but when you have a very bad head injury your only way to help the outcome was to properly ventilate, properly oxygenate the patient, and we must always ensure we maintain the mean arterial pressure (MAP) in the correct range. Over 75 or a Systolic over 110 as a minimum standard of care. So, think about it as the most important goals were to ensure adequate ventilation and adequate perfusion in order to maintain the brain function.

We also had to keep the mean arterial pressure up, which is the MAP. I knew even one episode of low BP meant death and a hypoxic brain was also death, so intubation and oxygenation was our first priority. Very soon after we got into the back of our unit, the other Tofield ALS crew arrived on scene and we went to work as a team. We had called for STARS right off the start. We had an IV access in a few seconds and then the bad news came: STARS could not come as they were already on a pediatric disaster call and it took priority as we could handle our mess. We also had the best available crews and we had the shortest transport time. We would double up our crew and have two medics in the back and we would save this kid, or at least try like hell. Losing wasn't an option. Not if any of us had any say in it and seeing as we all loved kids and had kids of our own, we would make her live.

It took three of us using the video laryngoscope and our experience but we got the intubation the first time and, just like that, we had the magical airway inserted and secured. From then on, it was easy street. Medications, monitoring everything from the cardiac monitors to the heart rate, the ventilations, the BP, the CO2 and the Sp02 for misadventures. Most of all we used diesel, which essentially meant we got the heck off scene and headed toward the trauma team as fast and as safely as possible. We had a plan and it was going to work. It had to.

Next up was a pelvic binder but as she was already scooped and it was not as easy. We did our best to bind her pelvis as it had to be broken. On the way to the city we updated the trauma doctors and the charge nurse at the U of A and they knew we were doing our best with what we had to work with. We could have used some mannitol, but it wasn't available. When we picked her up someone said she was twenty-eight but she looked like a kid. After we left the scene they told us she was fourteen and when we got to the trauma centre and they took her over, we realized then she was only twelve.

We could have used Dr. Broad as his suggestions would have been put to us in seconds. We elevated the head slightly as in head-injury patients, it helps decrease the intracerebral pressure (ICP), which is the intracerebral pressure, and in this case, it would be climbing. Nothing but a burr hole or mannitol would make any difference in such a bad head injury normally. Seeing as I had been shown how to do a three-finger technique to locate landmarks, I had an idea of how to do a burr hole. One very cool neurosurgery staff member I had befriended had shown me after we did one in the ER one night and had saved a life on a kid that was posturing. I knew I had his blessing but I was sure it was just a little out of my scope of practice. Plus, the local MacLeod's' Store that is now known as True Value hardware store was closed anyway so that wasn't an option. The only way to get her to the specialist was by us heading that way as fast as possible. It was a pure mercy mission on wheels.

En route her BP was around 220/180, which is not good. We just kept ventilating at the exact rate to keep the Sp02 at the correct numbers and kept giving the right medications to try to abort a brain herniation. Upon arrival to the city I was so glad to see the waiting trauma team. I remember walking into the U of A and seeing one of my past students and I was shaking my head. Sara Affolder, you were one of the best things I saw that night. Your eyes gave us hope when we had none left. I had no idea if this little one would make it.

I had never seen a patient have a BP this high and live. As soon as they took over, our job was done and I was so thankful that she was still alive despite the severe injury. Over the next several days the outcome did not look good but, slowly, she started to get better. Initially, they gave her no chance but in about four weeks she was trying to walk already and the rest is history. About a month after that, we got to meet with her and the other rescuers, she wanted to thank us for saving her life.

I have attended so many interesting and challenging calls in Beaver County over the years. As a team, we helped multiple people defeat their illness or injury. Multiple times we were called to assist in the local ER and helped to stabilize patients when they needed ALS. We were always blessed to work with the best dedicated nurses and staff doing what we did best on every shift that we could help. All in all, I never had regrets on our busy shifts. The best thing was no two days were ever the same.

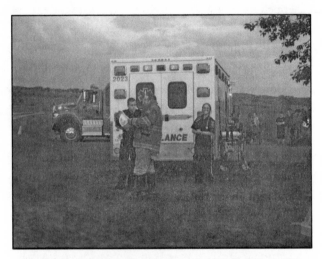

*"Saving Lives" "The Team Approach: Dispatchers – First Responders – Firefighters – EMS – STARS – Critical Care; everyone matters and everyone counts."*

# "In Harm's Way"

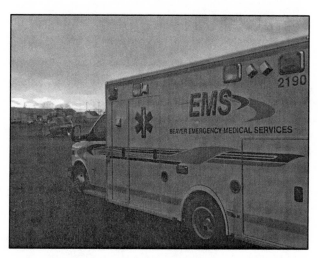

*"Doing Our Best"*

There are reasons we do what we do and my reasons are simple but multiple. I would have to state publicly that I'm not the person who I used to be, as I have evolved into a better person, thankfully, due to the influence of many. There are many influences in my life and many people who influenced me to become who I am today. The reason I care as much as I do today is because of the many people who helped show me the way. Somehow, after taking many wrong roads, I found the "right way" or the right path to my destiny. I might not be as good as I should have been or as good as I can be, but as the song from Tim McGraw, "Better Than I Used to Be," states it so well, especially in my case, that I'm better than I used to be. The people who helped me choose the right path in life are people I can't or won't ever forget. I will go over the main people and the important lessons that helped make me who I am today, giving credit where credit is due for the priceless lessons that I've so often learned the hard way.

The first person who taught me that caring was the right thing to do for everyone was Ann Marie Baerwald. Ann Marie was my best friend and taught me more than I can tell you. The most important thing that she taught me was that you can't pick or choose who to care for, as there are no bad people on the planet; some people had just made better choices than others. Ann Marie could always find good in others, and I'll always love her for that.

Allan Needham might have been but a farmer and a loner to many. But to me he was brilliant. Not only was Allan as strong as two men, he had many talents and was always helping others in times of need. I was so amazed at his wisdom and was always happy to call him a friend.

Next are the amazing Len and Evelyn Yates who ran the funeral home in Oxbow for many years. They had gone through hell on earth after losing their daughter to a drunk driver but always made the best of every day. For many years, they ran the ambulance as well as the funeral home. So, not only did they see tragedy on a daily basis, they also helped clean it up and had to go to work the next day knowing the pain and suffering many people never see.

Over my first number of years in EMS, I got to see people for who they were and not the disease or condition that they had or presented with on that day. That was incidental in many cases. The important thing was to treat the patient, as they mattered. When they were hurt, or had significant injury as well as presented with a medical illness, they were still a person. You would have to ensure you left your personal prejudices at home and disregarded how they might have gotten into the specific situation. They were human and you needed to be treated as you would treat a friend. I found that when they trusted you and you talked to them and not at them, you did better. If you communicated well with them, you sometimes needed to use less pain or sedative medications overall. They began to build trust in you and when you smiled, they smiled back at you even if they were in pain. I'd often joke with them and make light of the event even in very tragic situations, so they or their families would feel less worried.

There was a time to be serious but if you could keep everyone calm, it helped the situation out even more. Never make the emergency your emergency. You're the driver of the situation and you ensure your passengers are safe is a great analogy. Most times you are safe, but when you least expect it, trouble can come knocking, I found this reminder the hard way. I was laughing one second and not the next.

One time I thought I was totally in the right spot in the world and all was well. To think I was really close to getting shot or stabbed never crossed my mind at all. I had a night off from any worries and trouble was the least of my concerns. We were at the Wayside Inn and I was celebrating a good day to come tomorrow. In the morning, I was going to be married and a new chapter in my life would start. I was sitting with my back to the wall on purpose as almost every bar in town had its share of violence. I was joking with the two friends I was having a social drink with and we were all just relaxing after a tough week at work. We were just enjoying our time-sharing stories and making the best of a great night off.

We saw a small fight start out on the far side of the bar. In no time three local RCMP officers stormed right past us, as we were seated by the door. They went over to the fight and we could see them talking with some people but it looked like it was all over and that was that. In a minute, they were walking in our general direction when our night changed in an instant. I wasn't aware of time, just the knife coming out. The officer was going to get stabbed and I could stop it. Well, I would try and do my best and what happened would happen.

There was one RCMP officer walking ahead of the bad dude and two more police officers were walking a little farther behind him. The second officer I knew very well; Constable Ben Drapper had been a good friend of mine for years. Just as they got almost to our table on the way out the side door, I could see the knife come out of nowhere. I had no time to say or do anything but attack. I went straight for the guy's head and yanked his head backward so he couldn't stab the officer in the back. I got him by the neck as we all went down in a pile. Ben had also seen the weapon and had gone for the knife. It seemed like a completely harmless idea until the police officer leading the parade of people turned around and glared at me, and then I realized I was in serious trouble. I thought, "Okay, now I'm going to get shot." He yelled at me, "What the f--- are you doing?" I yelled back, "He's got a knife," and was waiting to get shot. Thankfully, the shocked officer figured it out before he decided to shoot me. After all, I did just save him from being killed. It would have been no good to get shot but if I died saving a police officer, that would be okay with me. But being shot wasn't what I had planned for the day before I was getting married. Plus, people had travelled from around the world to attend the wedding and I would be not very popular for not showing up. I guess it would be a memorable reason. I would have been missed, I'm sure.

There were many times in my life that my life would be threatened and I or the people I was working with would escape harm by some small miracle. There were a few times in my life that I was scared but I never had time to tell anyone. One night while working at the U of A in Emergency, I almost got more then I bargained for and it was truly an evil night in the making.

I was called to our D-Pod stat by our charge nurse. I was not security and was not supposed to help but I had the ability to help. With my size and my strength, I could move a truck if needed. I could do what I could do until they had enough security or the police could arrive. Before I even got close to D-Pod, I could hear the sound of breaking glass as I ran toward the problem. One very large crazy person was now naked and using a chair to beat the security doors down. He had already broken the first set of glass windows that were supposed to be shatterproof. He was now going to come out of the room and nothing but a bullet was going to stop him. No police were present and none in sight so I was basically on my own. Then it became too real as I started to look at the damage he had already created, and I got worried. I went into survival mode. He needed to be stopped before he started killing people. Not on my watch I thought. He would not kill my friends. Even if he was stronger and bigger then all of us, I would stop him or die trying.

The outer door hinges were bending. He was slowly getting free of his secure room one smash with the chair at a time. He had already torn the bed out of the solid mounts that held it firmly to the floor. I took one look at him and I knew if he got out, people would die. The city police were called but were not coming soon enough. The security lady was about 100 pounds, one hit and she would be smashed to pieces. I came up with a quick plan. I got someone to bang on the one door he was smashing down and distract him and when he looked that way I would go in the main door to his room and stop him. I just forgot to think it through all the way. I was going to stop him and that was it. Nothing else mattered at the time. I never thought about the glass everywhere on the floor. Good thing I had on my Superman shoes.

I thought it sounded like a good plan but I never thought about the glass all over the floor from the broken window pane. It was the only plan I could come up on short notice. My plan worked well for the first part as the entry was perfect. They distracted him beautifully. The little security guard had my back. Looking back, I'm sure it was over before she even got in the room. I went for him as fast as possible but I didn't realize he was so big, so I immediately launched myself at him and flew up about two paces before him. I hit him hard enough to take his head and top part of his body down backwards. In a split second, it was over. The fight was done. I didn't like to hurt anyone but I had to tackle him and win or there was no telling what he would do next. Nobody was going to die on my watch. Then the pain started to come to my brain. I realized I was hurt and that was not part of the plan at all.

When the room stopped moving, he was still down and I was still on top of him. This was when I realized my plan was flawed. My arm was under him and I found the glass that had cut my arm up. Crap, that was not the plan at all. In a short time, everyone else was in the room and took me off him and he was hauled away. Everyone was really worried about me and for a second I was not even aware if I was hurt or what happened. It all happened so fast I never saw it coming. He was taken to A-pod to get some sutures as he was cut up from attacking the door. Plus, he needed a time out.

I was kindly scolded by the charge nurse for getting hurt and taken away by my concerned friends. I got a free stretcher and a little time to rest and think about what just happened. That was when I realized I could have just been killed. Mel cut up my scrubs and got me all cleaned up and took away the extra glass I was carrying around. Then, one of my good friend's sutured me up and made me new again. I just needed a few weeks to heal up the physical scars.

It was not what I planned for that night but we had no other options. If he had gotten out I know someone would be dead. The chair was being used as a weapon and because of his huge size it was a losing match for everyone but me. Later on, I was reprimanded by management, but that was fine with me. The best part about it was they didn't have that much to go after me with as it was a pure self-defense issue. The videotape was reviewed but I never got to see it, thankfully, as I already relived it more than once in my mind.

Apparently, they could see a green blur go past the camera's field of vision and it was over. I never took it personally as they were management and I was just doing what I had to do to help my friends. If I'd died that night, at least I knew I'd have enough friends to act as my pallbearers and the wake would be a great celebration, minus me. I look after my friends and the people around me and I will always do the same thing. I was brought up to never look the other way. I would die for them and they knew I would come if they ever called me for help. Dave Trabish, Greg Siefert, Gary Lundman, Little John or any of my good friends would have done the same. Many other male nurses I worked with back then would have and continued to after I departed the U of A. My saving grace was that I was the size of a small truck hitting the train to derail it that night. I was the big man with the big heart and I knew I could do it even before it was done.

It was only my option and I would do it again. I just wish I had been a little faster. The incident happened on a normal Saturday night. The following Monday, the *Edmonton Journal* published his picture and his name and told people to be cautious around him as he was likely to reoffend. It said in bold letters, "If you see this man or have any concerns, please call the police TIPPS line directly." Someone had crossed out the TIPPS number with pen on the copy in our break room and put our number for the U of A ER which was 780-407-8832, and written, "Just ask for Dale."

It just took a few weeks for my arm to heal and I was as good as ever. I would never walk past that room again without thinking about the close call we all had. Gibbs' Rule # 44 fit the incident very well in my mind: "First things first: hide the women and children." They didn't want or need to see this large, crazy naked person try to kill me. It would have given them nightmares for years.

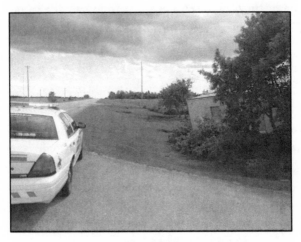

*"Police – RCMP - Keeping Us All Safe"*

# Dale's Rules: Points to Ponder for a Successful Career in EMS or Health Care

- *Be a true hero and accept your wins as well as your losses.*

- *Even with experience, knowledge and wisdom, we can be wrong.*

- *We will never always be right.*

- *We can't always win.*

- *Pay attention and learn from others' mistakes.*

- *We should not blindly agree with or accept everything we are told by people who are considered "experts." Everyone can be wrong sometimes.*

- *It's OK to agree to disagree sometimes.*

- *You could most likely count on one hand the times Spock was wrong, but he is not considered an expert, but a mere Vulcan.*

- *Gibbs is a great leader of the NCIS team, but he can't be expected to do the right thing every time. REMEMBER—LIFE DOESN'T LET US ALWAYS BE RIGHT.*

# "Ambulance Transport"

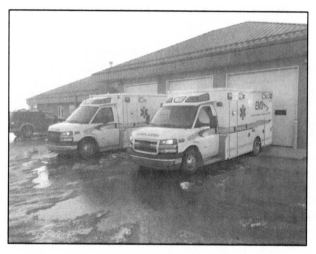

*"Doing It the Right Way"*

I would simply like to ask one question when it comes to the EMS world in general. Are we doing it right? Are we making a difference in all patient outcomes or should we be doing more or less? We frequently came across complex calls where it can be debated how much can be done by EMS and also how much should be done in the hospital setting. Every time I hear BLS is better than ALS or that the BLS providers can do just as much as ALS, I shake my head. I can't seem to make people understand that the higher level of care should be the bare minimum in all cases, even if you don't perform any ALS skills.

It's wisdom we should value. Too me it's the most logical to have an ALS level available or used when the situation determines the patient is unstable. As soon as you have any Level of Conscious (LOC) or low Glasgow Comma Score (GCS) problem, an airway problem, a breathing problem, and for sure if a circulation problem exists, BLS has exceeded their skill requirement level in many cases. It's best to utilize ALS early and have the highest level of care on all calls. One of the funniest calls I remember getting was when I worked in and was living in Lac la Biche and was called for ALS back-up. I was more than glad to come and help. On arrival, my friend was working hard doing his best and was more than happy when we arrived.

Charles was one of the BLS staff I knew well and I also knew he was more than competent. He had done a very good job. The oxygen was appropriate; the breathing was an adequate rate and depth. The vitals were stable. On the monitor, though, the rhythm was all over the place. I was seeing all types of different beats and it was not normal, but the patient was essentially asymptomatic as they had done the right interventions. I asked a few questions, got a detailed report and then I bugged the patient to ensure his brain was functioning well. If you can laugh, you're ahead of many people who are sick. I said, "Let's go to the hospital." Charles said, "Aren't you going to do something?" I smiled and said, "You've done everything that needs to be done. I'm just here today for moral support and if that heart rate becomes lethal or unstable, then I'm going to work." Just know that 'Do no harm' is the golden rule. On arrival to the hospital, the patient was happy and I think my role on the trip was doing what was right for that patient on that specific call.

But even to this day we see BLS crews cancelling ALS and transporting a patient in cardiac arrest with no extra hope in hell of living, all while smiling and being completely unaware they are wrong on so many counts. Just recently I was called with my partner for BLS backup for a witnessed cardiac arrest. The middle-aged man collapsed with his wife present and CPR was done immediately. The closest BLS was dispatched and we were the closest ALS, which was a long way from them, but considering they had no hospital close by we would bring the critical care to them. STARS would not routinely even be considered as this was often a futile effort, but we'd do our best just the same. Still, they'd said they could and would fly to a call if no ALS was available. So, I was thinking that we could always launch them if we got a pulse back. About halfway to the meeting point, BLS cancelled us and said they didn't need us and then they headed to a hospital, which wasn't even the closest hospital, which is the legal requirement, but they never followed that rule anyway. They actually went a different way so meeting us wasn't an option. I wondered if that was the plan all along, which made me even more upset, but no one cared so it wouldn't matter to anyone but me.

I ask you all: Why? Why not use ALS when you are only a BLS unit? I actually kept driving for some time and could have easily intercepted them, but we would be disciplined so in the end I just gave up. With my years of wisdom, I would say the BLS staff decided they were just as good as we were and they didn't need us. The end result, as you guessed, was a dead patient and, once more, I ask you: Did this really need to happen? I will keep fighting but when we keep questioning the decisions of certain BLS services and when they are supervised by BLS supervisors that have no insight or no wisdom, they not only doom the patients but hurt us all in the end. I hate losing any patients as they are so important to me and the reason I work so hard. If I did not care or was lazy I would be oblivious to the big picture. I should just forget it, but it still upsets me that our system allows stupidity to rule. In the olden days, we would have fixed this but the current system is so huge with so many managers that the loss of a few patients is not even a concern.

Very rarely do I get mad and if I do, there is a good reason behind it. On one call, I finally lost it and said exactly what I was thinking and no one said anything back to me as I was so right. We were sitting in Holden doing standby and one of the other communities on the east side was in need of ALS. As we were responding they cancelled us just before our arrival despite one dead ejected dog, despite one patient with critical injuries and despite the fact that one person was ejected and also visibly broken. But they didn't need ALS. I actually swore at the RCMP and the BLS crew on scene who thought ALS was over-rated.

Many times, we were tricked and told it was a BLS call but it was more like a holy crap call all the way to the hospital. One such call involved a woman with a bladder infection. It could easily have been just a BLS call. They even went so far as to make sure we didn't respond with our lights and siren on in the dispatch information. Well this one call will show you all the differences between the BLS approach and the ALS approach. I would have never expected the call to involve more than a simple transport to the local ER. But it turned out to be far from an easy call and made me think hard and fast. On this call, we would walk into the unknown, which is all too common in this profession.

On arrival, I parked on the street close to the house but not beside it. We decided to grab our basic BLS bag and we didn't need the monitor as it was just a bladder infection. A local police officer was on scene as well as he was just bored. We knocked and a family member took us to the patient's side. When I walked up to the patient to take a radial pulse and was going to start to joke with the patient, I was in for a shock. The joke was on me. Dispatch had specifically told us not to use lights and siren. The patient had a very slow, weak pulse and looked as if she was already in cardiac arrest. Her eyes were open but nobody was home. "Shit," I said out loud. We missed the chance to be ahead of the situation. I had to run back to the unit to grab our life pack monitor (Physio Control LP-10) and get it on the patient.

We could pace a heart from nothing to 140 beats per minute (BPM) in seconds or cardiovert a lethal narrow or wide complex arrhythmia. Sometimes we cardioverted someone with a synchronized cardioversion with as little power as 50 to 100 Joules, if we were lucky. But, commonly, when atrial fibrillation was the bad guy we needed 360 Joules the first time so it was wise to shock once at your highest power. The manufacturer claimed that it would convert about 89 per cent of the cases with 360 Joules. We just needed to ensure the patient was sedated first and correctly. I'd heard and still hear repeated stories of doctors shocking patients who are symptomatic but not unstable, patients who are wide awake with up to 360 joules being sent through their chest. It's inhumane but required if they are severely unstable, with no distal pulses and a GCS that is low. Words of wisdom: If they are unstable, use ketamine at the correct dose or a very low dose of a benzodiazepine and repeat it until they don't know or care you're around. You'll be much more likely to get a Christmas card instead of a death threat.

Well, this case today was a very unique challenge. I could see a strange junctional bigeminy rhythm. I can remember reading about how to treat it in one of my textbooks. This was called *Beck's Pharmacology* and was required reading for one of our Paramedic courses. I think it was on around page 93 and it said to try atropine and / or then pace it. Either way made sense to me. If that didn't work, then I could use Lidocaine as the last resort. Just think of it as the PVCs were causing retrograde conduction, which makes the messaging system not work right in the cardiac conduction system. If you treat the heart rate first and bring it up, the PVC might abort and then if it isn't effective, you treat the PVCs. This may sound easy but it was not as logical as it sounds. Spock would have said, "This is illogical." You never give Lidocaine for a junctional rhythm, normally. The problem that made me stop in my tracks momentarily was that this wasn't a normal textbook case. At the speed of light, I was thinking, "What are my options?" and in a mere second I had a plan. But the plan had its risks and risks were not what we liked when playing with someone's life. The patient was counting on us. The family was watching us and had everything to lose.

"Well," I thought, "I tried pacing and thought that should work but it didn't." Next, I tried atropine and still no change. By this time, she looked as if she was going to arrest. I was thinking it was almost time for good old CPR. I'm positive she would not have objected. Her family said to me she had arrested before with an arrhythmia but didn't know why. I thought we were heading there already. It was likely already too late today. But then I remembered what the book said and thought at this point I didn't have much to lose.

She was basically already in a pseudo-arrest already. I was watching the monitor and feeling for a pulse and then it hit me: the PVC were most likely causing the most harm. If we knocked them out, we'd win. If not, they'd win and she would die. I had to make a decision quickly. This was the part that sometimes you can get stuck on. It's always a risk-benefit ratio; your first and foremost rule is to do no harm. I could only use Lidocaine or magnesium and there was some rationale for using both. Lidocaine simply stabilizes the irritable myocardium and slows the messages that help with conduction but can block some good conduction as well as decrease the contractility effects somewhat. Magnesium is great for *torsades de pointe* or resistant arrhythmias and also good for malnourished patients. I had run out of time. I grabbed the Lidocaine and pushed it at 1 mg/kg and waited for the surprise.

Well, the pharmacology gods were on my side that night. In no time, the arrhythmia was aborted and we had a normal pulse, a BP that would easily sustain life. We got a shock as we transported and she became back to normal and stabilized. The ER doc gave me an evil look and the medical director who didn't particularly like me wrote me up. But all in all, I would have to say I was out of options. I could have waited until she died and tried CPR, or then tried Lidocaine as by then she would most likely be in ventricular tachycardia, which is one of the bad rhythms that can or may not have a pulse. But most likely she would have been in ventricular fibrillation and I would have shocked her with 200 joules and then she would have become asystole and died. By thinking hard sometimes you can come up with the right thoughts. Sometimes you will get the bear and sometimes the bear will get you. Today I saved the bear and now we will be friends for life.

Every once in a while, things happen that should not but they do in our patients and there is no logical reason. Not everything is written up in the textbooks. You will never have seen it all and if someone tells you they know everything in medicine, run away. It's a lie. They are uneducated in the real world of medicine. I frequently read medical books and research the new and wonderful aspects of medicine and it's amazing the new knowledge there is out there and still I can't read enough. But just know that medicine is always changing and evolving but often we return to old ways of doing a skill or intervention after people decide to change a current system. It was a lesson I learned in my lifelong EMS and medical career that things we did would always be changing. Many things we do are cyclical. They come and go with trends. So, after your next weird call, research the differential diagnosis and also the diagnosis. Really look at other perspectives and find out even one more thing that you didn't know before and you'll be better off than when you started your shift.

The ultimate call I want to share with you all is the call that proves that when we work as a team we save lives. I know we are in an endless battle of change and challenges but if we all work for the right reasons we become the team that nothing can stop. Even on a good or a bad day we can make a difference in others. One day I was doing what I do by enjoying life and had stopped at the local Wetaskiwin EMS office for coffee. We were enjoying sharing stories and laughing about our many adventures. I was sitting there visiting when a serious call came in. I grabbed a jumpsuit and minus my sandals, was dressed for battle. Sadly, it was only a medium size and I'm not a medium person. I could get the zipper up about halfway and that was about it. I got to respond with the Wetaskiwin EMS for the MVC that had become an MCI in seconds.

All we knew was that two minivans had gone head to head at highway speeds and we now had nine patients. It was going to big mess and everyone in the area was responding. STARS Air Ambulance was launched and would be coming ASAP. It was so positive knowing that we would have the best people trying to do their best to save as many as we could. But knowing the dispatch information, we were bound to lose patients as it was almost expected in these calls. You can't expect this type of accident to not have serious injuries.

On scene, I went to work and did what I could along with my EMS family members. We attacked with speed, with dedication and we made lives around us count for everything. In no time, I was starting IVs and getting drugs from any medic in sight as I had no narcotic pouch, as I wasn't really a paramedic that day, although I was much more than that in many ways. I would start an IV and push a healthy dose of morphine and then go to the next one. I think I did this to four people on my first attack. Behind me, staff were extricating and cutting people out. We had two teams with the Jaws of Life attacking the cars with vengeance. Doors were coming off. Roofs were being removed or laid over like a tin can, and all this in record time. There was no yelling or debating; it was a team of one and everyone was on the same level as we all were part of the team.

At one point, I was helping to remove a badly injured little girl and it made my heart break looking at her deep open lacerations across her face and head. She needed to be extracted and intubated. I would have cried if I had time but I had no time to cry. She was going to be one of the first to go in the STARS chopper and today we had more critical patients than ambulances on scene. As soon as we got her free I helped put her in the back of one of the MAA units. I was a little reluctant to just pass her over as I knew she needed so much care and Tim Essington, who was also my friend, could see my problem right away. He looked at me and said, "Dale, it's okay. Kevin has got this; he's a good man," and with that I jumped out and slammed the back doors shut and went after the next serious patient who needed my help even more then I could imagine. I had known Tim would ensure the patient was in good hands and I found out Kevin was just as competent as I was if not more. The little broken angel was in good hands.

I then found the one patient who needed my expertise in the worst way. She was on the verge of dying and was trapped in the front of the car with the front tire wrapped around her legs. She was barely awake but moaning and had no distal pulse anymore. I said to the fire crew to get out of the way as we had no more time to get her out the right way. They had been trying for some time but nothing was working as the van had molded around her legs and she was so broken but still trapped. I started to grab chunks of legs and just pulled hard. All of a sudden, the legs were freed. They resembled a pile of broken pretzels wrapped around each other. We had chunks of bones coming out the wrong way and the legs didn't even look human. It was just a mangled mess.

I used a great orthopedic trick and just grabbed the big toes and unwrapped the complete mess of her lower extremities and then pulled them both hard while supporting the pelvis structure. All of a sudden, the legs were back to an almost normal length and the multiple bones sticking out disappeared. Doing a pulse check was a waste of time as she had no blood left to make a stable BP so it wasn't a priority. We secured her to a spine broad and then it was time to get an airway, as when we extricated her we were losing it the same time we laid her down. Thank God, the STARS crew was landing at that time and Dr. Erica Dance, whom I had known for several years, was coming to my rescue and would assist me right away. I grabbed the last IV that I had left and there were no more as we had used them all up. It was a 16 gauge and was greater in size but in a hypotensive patient who has no BP left, it was not going to be easy to insert it. I just grabbed it and stuck it in the spot where it should work even when I knew the veins were essentially empty. But then and only then did I realize my mistake.

I had only one IV left and had grabbed it and put it in so fast that I realized afterwards that it was missing something important. I had left the Angiocath in the package and had just put the needle into the vein. I pulled it out and pushed the Angiocath on and stuck it right back in the same hole—and it worked. What I got was a small miracle as, yes, they do happen from time to time. I had never done that before and never will again. I started the lifesaving IV fluid into her wide open. Thankfully, she was so hypotensive that the bleeding was minimal but that wasn't a good thing normally. Next, we needed to perform an intubation and an advanced airway right now.

I had borrowed enough medications to help intubate her as she was still able to bite onto the airway and it would not be as easy as you would hope unless we sedated her or paralyzed her properly. The oxygen was blowing on her face and we were trying to enhance her preoxygenation as best as possible. I punched in the drugs as Dr. Erica Dance was intubating. Then I said, "Where is the BVM we just had ready to go?" A firefighter said they needed it to ventilate another patient. Crap, I thought. But we were right next to the Wetaskiwin Fire Department rescue truck and I had a Plan B. When I was a volunteer I had bought, and donated a BVM and it was on the rescue truck. I opened the door and there it was with the medical supplies. I quickly grabbed it and we were ventilating in seconds. We hardly missed a second but it was a close call. I told STARS they were getting a two-for-one deal today and they kindly looked at me and said, "Sure, why not?"

In the end, I left the scene with the last patient in a MAA mechanical backup unit. I was going to bypass and head to the city right from the scene and Tim said, "Dale, you can't." He was looking toward the cupboards. They had no supplies as they had been all used up that day. I could see his logic in bright colours and off to the Wetaskiwin Health Centre with a volunteer firefighter driving my unit I went, and we never looked back.

All in all, we had four patients with dislocated pelvises, we had done two separate rapid sequence inductions (RSI's) which are rapid sequence inductions to establish lifesaving airway with just the right medications. STARS took two of the critical patients from the scene and then did two more back-to-back flights to transport a total of six patients. They even had to get more fuel between the second and third flight, which is almost unheard of. We had done the impossible. We saved them all. I had to write five patient care reports PCRs, then testify two years later and never got paid a cent. But it was okay. I got a free coffee and the chance to help save nine lives, which was payment in full. It would be one of my busiest but coolest calls as I just did my job and nothing else mattered.

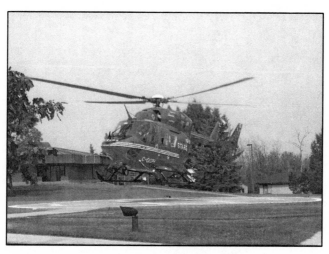

*"Saving Lives One Flight at a Time"*

## Chapter 22: *Making the Difference to Everyone*
# "You Matter"

When you ask me, what made the most difference in saving lives, I would have to say it was multiple components and never just one specific thing. The first part is the right people, the right partners at the right time and being at the right place. You need the right stuff—the equipment, medications and monitors. The right atmosphere sets the stage for success on so many levels. Finally, you need the right protocols or the right "On Line Medical Control" (OLMC) or critical care physicians as your backup for wisdom and support. There is also something to be said for fate or destiny. You can cheat on something in life but you don't cheat fate or change your destiny. If anything was missing, the odds would be against us in more ways than you can ever measure. We needed the right odds to win and the odds just weren't in our favour on some days.

One day we were called for a choking baby. The baby was 34 years old and was choking after drinking too much. He was walked to the unit and taken to the ER to sober up. We all felt a little relived but embarrassed as we were followed by an alert police officer who came as our backup, only to be told after we realized the "baby" was walking and talking that maybe we should slow done a little next time. He told me only two wheels were touching the ground on one corner. I asked him if it was the front two or back two. He didn't think that was funny.

Besides the pain and loss, I would witness on a regular basis, the worst part of the job was the prejudice I would occasionally witness or experience myself. Culturally, we aren't as diverse or as friendly as we should be in such a modern world. Even with the best medicine and the most unique diagnostic imaging we still mistreat people because of prejudices or because of misconceived ideas that cloud our judgment.

Many years ago, I was working in a very busy ER. We had one doctor who was Caucasian and prejudiced. When I questioned one of his orders as I frequently did, he told me that "I was the nurse and he was the doctor." I knew I was pushing my limits on many nights but I had to stand up for the patients. Some days we have to stand up to be heard more than others. I knew our patients were sometimes being discriminated against for who they were or where they come and it bothered me to no end.

One night the doctor said in front of the ER staff, "I'm getting sick of these natives." When he was told by one of our fearless nurses that maybe he should get a job somewhere else then, he was clearly unimpressed. Unfortunately, doctors often get away with things they shouldn't, as they are seen as godlike by many. This is the scary part when people need someone on their side.

One night a sick three-year-old came in with vomiting and diarrhea. He looked sick and was lethargic. I could actually smell ketones from the door of the room he was in with his mom. I told the mom not to worry, that would get him seen and treated and it would be okay. Unbeknownst to me, the doctor went into the room right after I walked out and told the mom she was abusing the emergency system and this child didn't need to be seen or treated. I was confused as I thought he looked sick and thought we should just treat him and make him better. It was an easy fix; we'd start an intravenous (IV) and give him some Normal Saline 0.9% solution until he could void, provide some Tylenol for his current weight and he would be better in no time. Kids get kick fast but also recover fast if they get the right medical help.

I went back to see the mom and give the child a needle as it was all I was allowed to do then. The physician had ordered me to just give the kid a dose of Maxeran, which was used for emesis and vomiting and then we were to send them home. I knew the doctor wouldn't listen to me as he had recently informed me all too politely that he was the doctor and I was nothing but a nurse. I really wanted to start an IV and give him a bolus or two and when he looked better, I'd send him home to be safe with his mom while he recovered.

But if I did that I would get in trouble. In the past, I had treated some people that needed it even if the physician refused or neglected to care and this was just another one of those times. I knew someday I would get caught breaking the rules and treating patients without an order even if the doctor was somewhat incompetent or not practicing wise medicine. I would then lose my licence.

I told the mom the doctor on call was an idiot and I could not change his orders. I told her I would leave a note for the next shift as there was a very good doctor coming on in about seven hours who would gladly admit her son. I knew he was sick but when I gave him the needle he cried a bit and I thought that was a really good sign. I reluctantly let them go home and expected to see them back later that day. The mom seemed okay with taking him home and I thought he would be okay if he stopped vomiting. I left a note for the day doctor who was well known to me and was always a team player and the night carried on. I just assumed the day doc would fix him as he was very good and all would be fine.

I finally went home at 7:00 a.m. after a long twelve-hour shift and was asleep in no time. When you're so tired you don't even remember driving home. Sadly, and tragically, the mom brought her son back in at 7:15 and he was in cardiac arrest. One of the nurses saw my note with his name and called me later that day to give me the bad news. They knew that I'd done what I could do and they, too, were devastated beyond words. The news broke me into pieces and even today I get upset and sometimes have trouble breathing when I think about it, and it's been over twenty years.

I couldn't sleep for days and days and I was broken beyond words. I had a son at home and he was the same age and looked a bit like the boy. They were about the same size and had the same build. They were also both the same on the inside with the same coloured heart and their blood ran red just like mine, but the other little boy did not receive treatment he needed as somebody in power had a dislike for Indigenous people and to this day I don't know why. I am certain that had he been white, he would have been treated and, ultimately, survived. But it wasn't the case.

On autopsy, he died from dehydration, which is very rare in the Western world. It was common in a third world countries with poor health care but Canada is far from a third world country. But it wasn't just dehydration and gastroenteritis that killed this little man. It was prejudice. I can't bring him back. I can't fix my mistake that night of not fighting hard enough for him. I never knew such prejudice and pain until that day. I wish I had treated him and lost my license.

Even worse, a few weeks later the same doctor was walking in the hallway in front of me and turned and looked at me and laughed. He said, 'I guess some days I should listen to nurses." I was shocked. I wanted to knock his head off right then and there. I hated this prejudiced doctor more than the worst criminal or lowlife I'd ever seen in my life. I reported him to the Alberta College of Physicians and this one rare time they listened. I testified at the hearing and had to look at his condescending face while he looked back at me like I was nothing for the whole trial.

I'm sure he hates me still. Thankfully, we got him out of town but not before he killed a kid who should not have died. One hundred years ago, dehydration would kill sick kids or children in Canada but in this day and age dying from starvation or dehydration in Alberta is beyond belief. The nurse that went with me for support to the trial later died from a self-inflicted overdose. It wasn't the only reason she took her life but looking back now, I'm sure it hurt her just as much as it did to me.

Over the next twenty years we would see a trend of increased scene times which corresponded with an increased mortality rate. It makes sense: if your patient needs an operating room then you should start to head in that direction ASAP. If you need blood or blood products for your patient then you should head to the appropriate hospital with blood or blood products. We always needed to plan our transports with the patient's care in mind. It would mean we needed to consider their present needs as well as the predicted needs during the transport. To be a rural paramedic we had unique challenges. We always had to consider our resources and also our transport times. I was always thinking ahead and some days it saved a life. One day in particular I was so fortunate to be stubborn. We were called to what sounded like a bad accident. They updated us that one victim was DOA, and next they cancelled us. I told my partner keep going; we were almost there, anyway.

Before we got on scene I thought about the mechanism of injury, plus the fact that there were two vehicles involved and nothing added up. I thought, "This is strange, as we know it's a bad accident and it sounds like one person was dead and yet they didn't want ALS." It was purely illogical. On arrival, the DOA was actually the critically injured man's dog. We parked close to the intersection and we saw it was one huge mess. A truck had gone through an intersection and struck a delivery truck. The truck's engine and transmission were on the road. The truck was mangled but still on its wheels. That driver was completely trapped as the truck had simply molded around him.

The delivery truck had its box ripped off and its cargo was spread everywhere. The driver had been thrown and was lying beside his truck and was also injured. It was as if a bomb had gone off as there were parts everywhere. The dead dog was in the middle of the mess. I parked and went up to the first truck and there was an EMT and a police officer standing by the truck. I asked what they had. "Two patients," they said and one as awake, which is why they cancelled ALS. I still think this is why people die more often than they should;

the system is so top heavy and the workers have no idea of what they can or should do. It was a common problem.

That was the second I lost it. I said to them both, "What asshole cancelled ALS?" I quickly grabbed my cell phone and pushed #4567, which was the direct link to the STARS helicopter crew's dispatcher. I just said, "If these assholes cancelled you, don't listen to them. Get over here ASAP." I was really mad. I turned back to them and made a plan with my partner to set up for an RSI and IVs and once we could get the guy out, we would try to save him. The BLS crew was going to package the second victim and I told them to start IVS and head to the closest hospital.

I knew our patient was broken by quickly assessing him, but he was awake, semi-alert and his airway, breathing and pulse were present and relatively stable. His injures could be stabilized and, if needed, STARS could make a second flight and bring him back to the city as he was going to need an urgent orthopedic consult in my humble opinion. The other guy wasn't so lucky. Fire was on scene and starting extrications.

We had police and county police present and the roads for all directions had been shut down. We couldn't do anything to the patient who was still trapped in the vehicle as we were at a loss, to even touch him for a long time. After about forty minutes we could see and hear STARS as they made their final approach before landing. It was only then that we gained access to our patient. Time was against us. The fire crews had been cutting and extricating the vehicle off the patient and it took time.

As soon as we could, we performed an emergency extrication and had the patient in our unit. The other patient had been packaged and was already en route to the closest hospital. Additional ALS members had arrived and elected not to go with the first patient and BLS ended up taking him on their own without the benefit of ALS. That was not my idea. It was out of my control as we had our own problems to deal with.

As soon as we got our patient into the unit we learned the bigger picture. Bilateral flail chest, hypotensive with intraabdominal injures and all his extremities were broken. We got one quick IV but lost it when STARS got into our unit. Then it was intraosseous injection (IO) time. We had a special drill that would drill into the bone and it was performed by the STARS medic on their arrival. It was our life saving lifeline to administer IV fluids and medications. It was also medication time for we needed to sedate and intubate our patient for his flight in the STARS helicopter.

The patient was adamant that I look after his dog. I said, "Sir, don't you worry. As soon as STARS takes you, I will look after your dog. Sadly, his dog was ejected from his truck and was laying in the middle of the wreckage. I understood his concern as I had two dogs as well. I'm sure it was his best friend. I told him one more time just to make sure he understood and then he settled off to sleep. I said, "Don't you worry, I will look after your dog." It was a promise I had to keep. I kept my promise.

We gave him some perfectly compounded medications and he went to sleep, then we intubated on the first attempt and we also performed bilateral chest decompressions. The IV fluid was running wide open and off to the STARS helicopter he went, still alive, despite the mess. I was still angry about the fact that BLS had said ALS wasn't required. We had done our job and we packed up and left the scene as quickly as possible. Then dispatch was on us again for responding as they'd cancelled us, and I got mad all over again. I told them to disregard the cancellation, that we were needed and used despite people with a lower IQ trying to cancel us. Life was precious and to let people die was not something I could sit by and let happen, so I would take the flack for that, too. Then when we got to our base, I got another reminder to follow the rules, which I would take into consideration.

It was hard for me not to say, 'You're a bunch of idiots and you just failed the ALS and Critical Care Requirements test," but I shut up. It's just one of Dale's logical rules and it is easy to remember. If you have an Altered LOC or an ABC problem, ALS is your friend. Think: ABC

– or – LOC (Problems) = ALS). Later on, I heard our man survived about six weeks in ICU and then slowly recovered despite him not needing ALS. I guess they missed that one on NCIS, which was Gibbs Rule #15, "You always work as a team." It's the team that saves lives and not just an individual. Everyone matters.

That call was very hard but in the end, we got it right the first time around. We made a difference despite the problems we encountered. We helped do the impossible many times over and over. We made the team better by working as one and that was mandatory. We made the worst days for people a little better. Many days I would be pushed to my limits and sometimes, a little too far, it would seem. I would somehow come across an angel who was sent to help me when I needed it the most. I was blessed with a few guardian angels who would appear out of the blue to help me in times that I was in trouble, mentally and also spiritually. To Dr. Samina Ali, you will always be special to me. They say one person has the ability to save a life and you and Rena Sutherland sent me a message when I needed it the most. Our friends are the reason we can get back up and fight when we have nothing left.

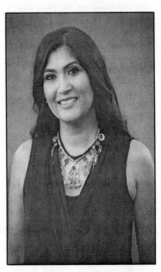

*Dr. Samina Ali, Pediatrician, U of A – Stollery*

# "PTSD, Compassion Fatigue and Stress Management"

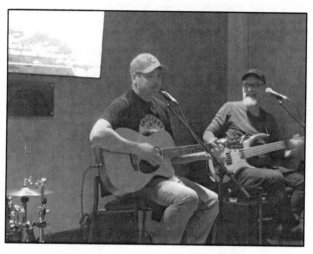

*"Kevin Davidson—LIVE—Making a Difference*

I would suggest strongly we need to address post-traumatic stress disorder (PTSD) and stress management better than we have in the past. No one else should die by their own hand as these are preventable deaths. We have also seen too many good people turn to alcohol or drugs to take away their PTSD pain. If we could just help the suffering deal with their problems up front and save even one life in the process, it would be worth it.

The first and most important thing I can say about our EMS family is the dedication we have to our partners. When I look back, I can count a few partners that made me a better person. I will share with you a few of them with you and after I'm done, you will see a different side of me.

Ann Marie and I were partnered up a long time ago but I can never forget the lessons she taught me. The biggest lesson was that everyone is special in their own way. Ann Marie was diagnosed with cancer and, before I knew it, she was gone. Many people will never know how special she was in my heart. We did a few tragic calls together and it was so nice to know we could talk about the pain and suffering we had seen and what was bothering us without having to worry about looking weak. She will always be one of the most sincere and caring people that ever walked this earth and the world lost one incredible lady and a great RN/EMT-A the day she left us.

Many years later I would come across Troy Harnish. Now here was one cool, educated dude with so much life experience. Troy was one of my students and we were a lot alike. Slowly, we grew a special bond that is rare among the students and instructors. We ended up keeping in touch after graduation and when he started flying air ambulance missions in the Northwest Territories, I was so happy to see him come to the University of Alberta Hospital – Stollery with his patients. It was common to see him coming through the doors at Triage with the ventilator set just right and four or five infusions running, smiling all the way to the ICU or the CCU. On a scale of one to ten, as a paramedic he was definitely a ten in my books.

Troy always went above and beyond the basics and ensured the patients had the right care and the right medications were given at the right doses to ensure the patients' outcome would be optimal. After good calls, he would text me and after hard calls he would text me. It was common for me to get texts from many students after graduation, asking about the best care options while running a code or seeking an expert opinion in a hurry when time was not on their side. If I didn't have the answer, I had contacts that did and we would do our best to help them out. Then after a few bad calls, things went to hell for Troy in ways not imaginable to most.

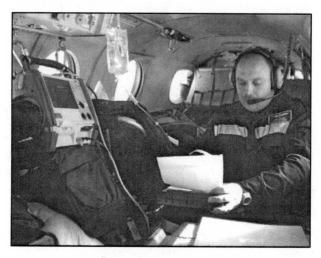

*"Troy: Giving Your ALL"*

Most people will never know the feeling of helplessness in a plane flying over the middle of nowhere with no one to help, when all hell is breaking loose around you and you're losing another patient and fate is against you. Destiny was likely already decided before the medevac mission ever started and that is why you were called. I know and have seen that hell before and it still haunts me. Before I knew it, he was back home, on leave from work, beaten and broken and had nowhere to go but up. Troy was in survival mode but due to PTSD, he was unable to work and no one cared or was willing to help him. Basically, he was a lost soul and it was up to him to get out of his ordeal on his own. Tragically, I was unaware of most of this and Troy, being a proud person, never said anything. He just went on day to day and was getting nowhere and was slowly losing the battle. When I found out, I was shocked and I called him right away. My heart cried for him that day.

I would have never realized how bad it was until one day in March 2014, I was reading the postings on Facebook and was shocked to see my friend's backhoe up for sale on Kijiji. I thought "He needs that backhoe—what is he doing selling it?"

I had no idea that the Workers' Compensation Board had cut him off from any support and he was losing the battle of his life. I talked to my friend Nathan, and in no time, I had a plan of attack; I would not let him lose everything.

Until recently, we had not heard much about PTSD, but looking back I had three or more of my former students take their own life. Several nurses and several RCMP I knew had also died by suicide and it made me wonder what was going on. I didn't know until I started to research it more that PTSD is extremely common among EMS workers, as well as those employed in the medical field and the military. I was shocked to see the numbers are even more dramatic among physicians, dentists and respiratory therapists. One article I read said that the US loses about 400 physicians a year and one small community lost seven in just one year. This was the worst of the worst news I could ever think of. The condition was killing too many of us and for so many reasons. But ultimately it all goes back to us caring for others and caring too much in many cases.

I was shocked but not totally, as I knew I'd had my own issues after bad calls but didn't understand it very well. After reading lots, I realized it's been a problem since the beginning of time but hasn't been very well understood. Almost everything from alcoholism to burnout to acute psychosis could be attributed to PTSD, but still no one was talking about it. If you had it, you were weak, or you were simply burned out. I knew this was not the case.

On August 3, 2015, a coworker, Shanna Renee, and I decided to organize a short walk to raise awareness for EMS personnel with PTSD. We walked around Viking but stayed close to our unit, in case we had an emergency call or a transfer. It took us ten hours to walk 50 km. It was an amazing day for me as it showed me that I could do much more than I thought if I just put one foot forward after the other and never quit. I was so proud of my friends. We also had Constable Bye checking up on us throughout the day. Mike is another amazing person whose wife is one of Paramedics with Beaver EMS. A great, small family that supports each other after their own bad days all while raising a family.

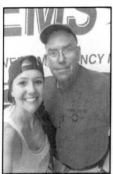
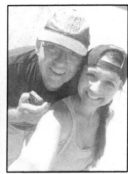
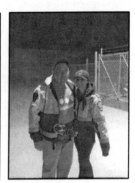

## Walking for PTSD (Shanna/Dale)

Now, I thought, what else could I do for Troy and how could we fix or make his life better? When Nathan suggested starting a GoFundMe account, I had no idea what that was so I started to research it. In a few hours, I had it set up. I started emailing my friends for help. In sixteen months, we raised just over $15,000.00. I will always be so proud of my friends for stepping up and making it possible. It made me realize that we mattered to so many people. I wanted to prevent another of my friends from killing themselves. If we even lost one person we would lose a part of us all. We stopped the GoFundMe program short of our goal of $50,000 since Troy didn't need it as he had a disability pension coming in. We'd done enough to make his life better and that was what counted the most.

My next goal was to show support for all the people we were working who suffered from PTSD. We organized another walk and in just over a twenty-four-hour period we walked approximately 100 km. I even had to stop for a bit in the middle of the night and help intubate a patient in the local ER. At 5:00 a.m. they had a vehicle malfunction so all the equipment had to be transferred over to the other unit and I had to help with that as well and then continue walking.

During the next day, we headed toward the small town of Kinsella. This was our planned halfway point. On the way back, we were hit by driving wind and pelting rain that tried to stop us but we kept going. It may have slowed us down but we never quit. All the while we picked up support from our friends on Facebook, and people passing us honked and waved at us. We showed people suffering with PTSD we cared about them and that we had seen and felt the same pain they have.

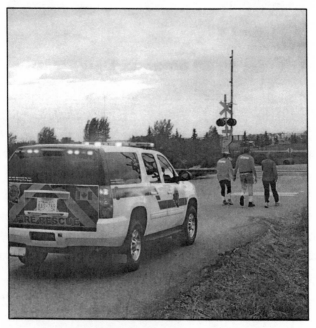

*"100 KM and One Huge Challenge"*

We raised some money that first year and at the end of the walk we had a great barbecue sponsored by our management at Beaver EMS, as well as some help from the Viking Fire Department. It was so unreal walking into the barbecue with so many people standing and clapping and cheering us on.

That night after the walk I was exhausted, sore and needed to go to sleep. It was just a few days before my fiftieth birthday and I had pushed myself harder than I thought possible.

Looking back, I think I walked 343 km the month before the walk. I had planned to sleep the day before the walk but instead I spent ten hours doing emergency calls so my little rest before the walk was cancelled. The walk showed us all that we could do it and that we stood as one. It was an amazing feat. It will always be one of my greatest personal accomplishments.

The next year I was started planning the walk early and we had picked May to make it coincide with EMS Week. We were going to make it better than last year until bad luck found me. Five weeks before the walk I hurt my right ankle and foot very badly, responding to a cardiac arrest call. I was running down a flight of stairs and something happened at or near the bottom of the last stair, and I was done. I went to the code, which turned out to be false alarm, and then I went straight to the ER for a splint or a cast not realizing I need more than a cast or a splint. I worked the rest of the night with an ankle that was very angry and kept swelling, despite ice, elevation and a tensor around the splint.

I was so upset at myself. I would never be able to walk 100 km this year and I would be lucky to walk a third of it. I was in a Robo Boot for a few weeks and could barely walk at all for a month. Some people said just cancel it but I refuse to do that. We needed to show others in EMS that they mattered. Hurt, broken, in pain or crawling, I wanted to and would make it happen. I was at physio in Sylvan Lake three times a week, in a Robo Boot and trying to get better fast. When my therapist Jen said I wasn't going to be able to walk it, I cried. But I knew she was right and as it stood from my MRI results I was in big trouble.

If I wasn't careful I would not be able to walk normally ever again. Many times, in physio, I was in so much pain that I came close to passing out. Jen was so amazing in many ways. She got to know who I was, what I did for a living and why I pushed so hard and she was on my side every step of the way. She learned things about me while I was having my treatments that I have never told anyone else.

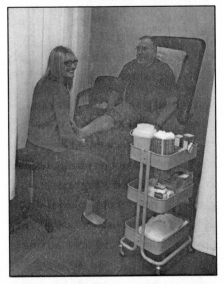

*"Physiotherapy works: Jen making me better, one treatment at a time."*

I knew after talking to Jen that I was completely wrecked and that walking even ten or fifteen kilometres wasn't realistic at that time. Then I had an amazing nurse, Nicole Lehr, from the Wetaskiwin General Hospital (WGH), contact me and say she would push my wheelchair. I also had a few other friends step and say they would walk for me. It actually made me cry. We were going to make it happen.

My son Evan would drive the support vehicle for me and my daughter Robyn would also walk some of the distance, as well. Plus, Tammie Dale and Jennifer Roadhouse had said they would be there and that was what I needed to get off the ground and make it work. I knew we could do it after Nicole and the others committed to me and my support team. My friends were not going to let me down; they were the ones who would carry my spirit and we would do it as a team.

Another great lady had also contacted me. The previous year, she had walked across Western Canada for a PTSD and SSPT organization. Kate Mac heard I was broken and got her rucksack out and knocked the dust off it and was coming to support me. In the past, I had seen her at the University of Alberta and helped her when she was severely injured in a parachute jump gone wrong. It was overwhelming to me to see the support from such an amazing lady who had seen hell and survived.

A few days before our planned walk, Fort McMurray was devastated by the huge fire. Kate then committed to her family and friends to load up a trailer with emergency supplies for as many people as she could help. But standing in her wings was one of her best friends, Mike Koestlemaier. He'd agreed to stand in for her and he did much more than that. Mike not only walked, he led us all until we reached Ryley then he took a rest to let the rest of us catch up. Mike was our hero.

The walk was attended by more people this year and I was so glad the Alberta Paramedic Association group supported us and came and participated as well. We took turns walking and this year we walked from Kinsella to Tofield. We had about five of us who walked most it. The leader for the majority of the walk was Mike, who is ex-military and could march and walk without taking breaks or resting. He volunteered to support our cause for EMS even though the military is well versed in the battle with PSTD, as well, and he was fighting the battle himself. With Mike in the lead, followed by Nicole, Louise, myself and a few others, we were off. The blisters were many but the bonds and friendships we created were forever. We raised over $5000.00 so overall it was a huge success.

Next year we may have to change the walk but regardless we will do something and we will do it together for PTSD awareness and also to raise awareness of Compassion Fatigue. It affects us all and all at different times: birthday parties, while shopping in a busy mall . . . funerals get me the most and I can't go to them anymore. Some people are affected most when the situations are similar to ones they've experienced at work, which can involve sounds, smells, feelings and odours unique to injury or death. I had been part of the code team that worked on a gentleman who had his liver blown out with a rifle. The smell of liver takes me back to that call almost every time I smell it. We will do what it takes to keep our EMS family alive and out of harm's way. I will and do take on other people's grief to make their day more manageable. That's why I am who I am and it's my chosen job.

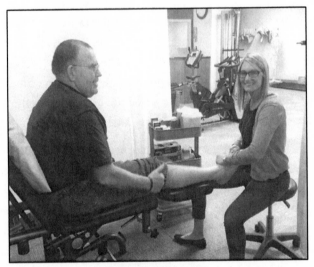

*"Making Me Better"*

Somehow, someway, we will beat this PTSD and show each other we can count on each other even if the system doesn't take time for us to recover. We will watch one and other's backs 24/7. After we lost a coworker and fellow student, Greg Turner, a paramedic from Edmonton who took his life after a series of very bad calls, I was flooded by messages that came in from nurses, doctors and EMS staff with whom I'd worked over the years. So many of the messages made me break down and cry. We can't save Greg as he's gone, but we can save as many as we can in the days to come. Even if I just help to save one person's life, it's worth the effort.

Over the last several years the sound of music has saved me when nothing else seems to help. By using music therapy and playing songs that mean something to me to get through my shifts. It's common for me to put on some music and listen to it all shift in ICU/SCU, as you're there almost all night by yourself. Music is very therapeutic. It can take you to the traumatic events in the past and bring you back again in some magical way.

My other saviours are my golden retrievers. No matter how bad my shift is, when I come home they are ecstatic to see me. All they want is affection and love. What therapy options do you know that provides that day in and day out? Some of my worst days they have held my broken heart and put it back together. After you've seen the amount of pain and suffering as many of us do, it makes you different. It's not burnout. It's more likely a combination of Compassion Fatigue and other complex issues. Lack of sleep, bad dreams, nightmares and thoughts of pure bad events make it very difficult to be productive.

The best way to recharge is to be around good people. Looking back when we thought we were helping one person, we touched many others at the same time. When Troy was in trouble and at his lowest point in his life, his partner was trying to keep everything going. I know that if Troy was hurt or hurting, Bonnie was also hurt. Many never consider the fact that it's not just the person with PTSD who suffers, their family and those surrounding them suffer, as well. So, when we helped Troy out of his mess, we helped Bonnie at the same time.

Bonnie was doing everything she could to keep them both afloat. Bonnie was right at Troy's side when he was beaten and broken to little pieces. Then when the worst of the worst was over, Bonnie stayed. When they decided to complete their vows, and get married, everyone could see Bonnie had a new light inside her and every day that followed, the light shone brighter.

On their wedding day, I've never seen a happier person in the world. We helped Bonnie as much as we could and in time I would see the rewards in triplicate. From the first time I had met Bonnie, I could see that we had helped someone who was a truly amazing lady who was 110 per cent dedicated to Troy.

Troy had the best hiding place in the world facing the ocean that is only accessible by quads or a Navy SEAL team, I would suspect. The location has a spot you can sit and just watch the ocean and the world go by and feel safe. It's an isolated cove off the south side of the Bay of Fundy where you can just sit and listen to the sounds of the ocean, the waves and the occasional bird flying overhead.

You can almost see Digby, Nova Scotia, and the Maine coastline to the southwest. When I was out there visiting Troy and Bonnie, we toured New Brunswick, Nova Scotia and spent a few days in PEI. New Brunswick will be where I retire one day. This vacation I took at Troy's was my way of recharging and my PTSD therapy. Some of the best therapy in the world is spent on a quad by the ocean at low speed while wearing a helmet.

I have seen many terrible things in my line of work—the things that nightmares are made of—but the reward has been the people I've met along the way. They have cancelled the evil or badness I have seen.

There is a saying that goes, "The closer you are to heaven, the farther from hell you will be." I surround myself with friends who are humble, caring and who bear no prejudices toward others. I may not be able to change destiny, but I sure as hell can fight the good fight along with my friends in this life of caring and helping others.

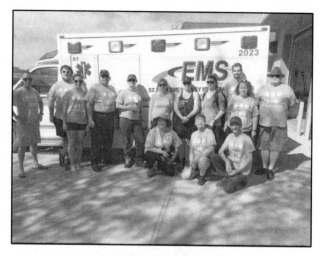

*"Walking for EMS, 2016"*

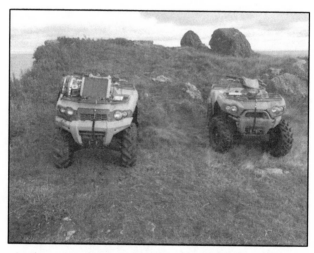

*"By the ocean: defeating PTSD my way."* Ray making the
best of riding the quad to the ocean in New Brunswick.

# "Doing Our Best with the Best"

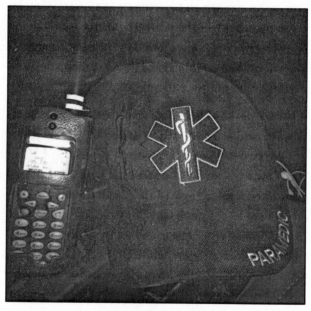

*"Giving 110 percent"*

There are times you have to ask yourself why some people live and why others die. I have seen accidents where the damage to a vehicle is about $500.00 with fatalities on scene and some where the damage is around $50,000.00 and no one was hurt bad enough to transport. This is before first generation or second-generation airbags. I strongly believe if you are meant to die that nothing we do right or wrong will change that fate. Fate is determined by a much higher power then our gifted hands.

We can help the odds or hinder the odds some, but if you have the will to live from within and the right people are praying or wishing for your success, it can defeat the devil's chance of taking you prematurely. The thought that I have saved so many lives in my career is not there, for I know I saved some by my actions but I made thousands comfortable with my words of encouragement, my tender therapeutic touch and just the right amount of medications from my drug box. Over the years, the medications changed but the therapeutic responses were found in the right combinations on many occasions. You could never give too much affection or pay too much attention to your patients.

One of the hardest but best paramedic calls started just like so many. It was a cardiac arrest with an unknown history on our initial dispatch. We arrived shortly and found a wife doing CPR and even more shocking to us was the fact that the wife was a nurse I knew and had worked with in the past. It was all the more reason to do our best and not let the devil win this time. We quickly took over the CPR and backup also came from the city police. The next biggest problem was an airway from hell itself. Every chest compression brought more fluid into the already blocked airway. There was literally fluid running out of our patient's mouth as we were doing CPR and we were unable to clear the airway. I was thinking back to the sickest patients I had seen and this never happened in any of them this badly ever. Today would be a new lesson in saving lives but I needed to get ahead of the worst outcome that would take another life.

I had attempted a few intubations after suctioning, but as soon as I went to pass the endotracheal tube, the airway was already full of water. Crap, I thought, and switched to Plan B right away. I took the suction and shoved it into the base of his throat and let it keep suctioning all while I was intubating. This time I saw the vocal cords and the tube slide past the magic opening and we were good to go. Inflate the cuff and ventilation was now possible, all while doing continuous chest compressions. Despite his being in cardiac arrest, we were golden. We had an airway and we could ventilate. The next problem was refractory ventricle fibrillation, which we shocked into asystole. Then post shock I gave him epinephrine 1 mg IVP and atropine 1 mg IVP, for which he went right back into ventricular fibrillation. Then this cycle repeated itself one more time. Time to change the attack pattern and come up with a better alternative, I thought.

I was thinking hard and I had a thought from my past reading into difficult cases. I remembered the Europeans had an approach that was unique and had proven successful. It was stacked shocks of 360 Joules as fast as possible followed by CPR and/or lidocaine, if available. We had been into this arrest for a long time. It was time to make a difference or we would lose the battle and time wasn't on anyone's side today. Therefore, I gave the lidocaine 100 mg IV and immediately shocked him three times as fast as the machine could go. It worked right away. We had a pulse and just like that, we had a life back.

We had beaten the odds for at least a minute. We quickly packaged and initiated transport to the local ER and we had STARS down beside us in no time as our backup as well. They took over the call and transported the patient to the local ER. My partner and I went outside the hospital and took a minute to catch our breath. We looked at each other smiled and laughed and hugged each other. We had faced bad calls before and won and lost a few as well. But today we beat the odds big time. We went back to make sure he was still alive and he was now stable and ready to fly away to a better place—but not with the angels, we thought. Looking back, he had defeated death twice. Thank God, we went the extra mile for him and made the effort to do what it takes to save a life. We never quit, nor did his spirit to live.

The next day I stopped by the CCU and went to see how he had made out. Well, I walked into his room and he looked right at me. Then I was shocked when he talked to me, as well. Extubated, with a hoarse voice, I'm sure, from the difficult intubation, but amazingly alert, awake and, most important, a save for us all. To be in a cardiac arrest for so long and now talking and able to thank us for saving his life was truly amazing. I remember his wife giving me a big hug with a few tears and I knew we had done the right thing.

Looking back, this was one call where paramedics made a difference and BLS would have lost the battle before they started. This is a big part of why we all need to work as a team and help each other along the way. Everyone needs to work together and make sure we look after all our patients the best we can. When we do that, our patient care is improved and our patient survival rate increases.

I was working in SCU/ICU by myself all night and always keeping a watchful eye on my patients. Lois would agree my paperwork sucked somedays but my patients were always clean and comfortable, or I was on top of the problem like a parent looking after a sick child. This one day I had a very nice man who kept passing out. His wife was a little upset with him as he had passed out a few times and kept smashing his face into hard objects, mostly in the bathroom. He looked like a serious case of elder abuse. I would have sworn somebody didn't like him and every time he came around the corner someone was hitting him with a large stick. But he said abuse was out of the question. Sometimes a patient's history is everything.

Our doctors in the ER were amazing. They had worked him up very well. His vital signs and 12-lead were done, as well as a complete laboratory investigation, which was normal. They even did a computerized tomography (CT) of his head due to his repeated head trauma. This was in order to rule out a cerebral event causing the person to pass out or become unconscious. We would try to rule out a bleed, such as an epidural hematoma or even a new subdural bleed. He didn't present as an alcoholic so the chance of finding an acute on chronic subdural was not likely. Basically, he was admitted for us to watch for an arrhythmia or a reason why he kept having syncope episodes.

We often admit patients with a suspicious history and look for a reason such as a heart blockage or tachycardia, which can be lethal or just problematic. Every once in a while, we would come across something that was not clear or we had no idea what was wrong with the patient other than that something was not right. Sometimes it was simply an abnormal presentation or a suspicion about the cause of a syncope or even a sudden cardiac arrest event. Most cardiac arrhythmias were not bad or lethal but they made the patient symptomatic, which makes them dizzy, feel faint, or gives them chest pain with or without some shortness of breath (SOB). Rarely these symptoms come out of nowhere and create some instant havoc unless they are ventricular fibrillation or pulseless ventricular tachycardia. These are the cases when having an AED or EMS close by to defibrillate your heart is lifesaving.

All night I watched the patient like a hawk and he was fine. We joked about his predicament. He laughed and we had lots of fun that night. I bugged him just like I bug everyone. I would often tell my patients in the SCU / ICU to just follow my most important rule and we would get along just fine. It's a simple rule: "Don't die." Near the end of shift, I was busy with one of my other patients and I was always watching out of the corner of my eye for problems with the others. You always listened to your monitors and you never knew when someone would push a Code Blue button, so you were always a little on edge. Suddenly I watched this guy just go backwards on his bed from a sitting position. I knew something was wrong but I couldn't see his monitor and didn't have any clue as to what the problem was just yet.

I immediately quit what I was doing with the other patient and walked past my desk so I could call for help. As I walked past the desk, I grabbed the phone and pushed the speed dial button for the ER and said to one of my good friends, Becca, "Help," and hung up. They were my best backup 24/7, or if it was really bad I'd just push the Code Blue button, but it was a little less discreet. That would wake up the world. I didn't think it was needed just yet.

As I was walking past my desk I noticed an asystole on the monitor display. This was not an uncommon problem if the patient pulled off his EKG monitoring leads. We usually didn't worry about it if the person was talking or we could see active breathing signs. But "Houston, we had a problem today," I thought.

I got to his side in a few long strides. I took one look at him and I knew he was in cardiac arrest. After many years of coming face-to-face with death, you get to know the look. I had a quick feel of his neck and wrist, and as expected there was no pulse, but he still had some ineffective breathing which meant it was a conduction problem. He was just looking forward at nothing with his eyes open and no one was home. This was too good of a man to lose this way, and I knew this was past being serious about ten seconds ago. I wanted him to live long enough to fall out of his rocker and die of old age. Thankfully, it was backwards on his bed, so his wife would never get the blame for this one event.

I positioned myself for chest compressions and thought about his history and why this had happened all too often to him. In the past, he had always hit the ground and woken up despite having new bruises. So, what if I waited and gave him a few more seconds and saw what might happen when his heart has some time to reprogram itself. I waited and was cursing myself for not pushing the Code Blue button. I knew cardiac cells have the ability to make a beat from anywhere in the heart as the tissue is proarrhythmic and would make a beat even if the SA or AV node was on strike. Then, all of a sudden, he came back and his eyes started to get life back in them. It took about forty seconds of nothing and then his conduction system said it was time to get going or he would just die. In seconds, everyone was surrounding him and we had declared war on his bad heart condition. We attacked him with treatments and we were not going to let him leave the planet just yet.

We had the pacer pads on and ready to take over if needed; lab had done another 12-lead. We also got the medication ready to sedate him and the right equipment ready as well as the staff ready to intubate him if needed. Our wonderful ER doctor then called cardiology and we had him ready to leave for an urgent pacemaker in record time. Thanks to Dr. Bakshi for coming to my rescue in seconds as well as a few of the best of the best ER nurses.

We had a plan ready if his heart stopped again with a Plan B and a Plan C. Then we did something I'd only done once in my career before today but had rehearsed over and over. It was not a common treatment suggested by the cardiologist on the phone and it made me laugh as it was not used very often but effective just the same. It was that we start an Isuprel (isoproterenol) infusion to maintain a faster or stable heart rate. Essentially, we could make his heart beat chemically faster than normal but could also make it a little bit more irritable so it was not straightforward. It was used on heart transplant patients or patients who had a denervated conduction system. We titrated the infusion rate up to the right dose to keep the heart rate faster than normal. Cardiology had booked him for a pacemaker in the next two weeks on his admission, but this event got him to the top of the list right now and today was the day.

My only caution to everyone is simple and concrete wisdom. If we start to not care, we are not therapeutic. If we are not therapeutic, we become the problem. When we become the problem, our patients—especially the ones with special needs—suffer. Helping others is an art and also a little bit of being a mad scientist, as no two problems are corrected in the same manner. Sometimes everything goes right but sometimes we keep failing and need to be more creative in our solutions. The more you know in medicine, the more creative you can be as long as you're ensuring that you're not making the problems worse.

Someday you will just do something and in the end, you will see it made the difference that day. It's called instinct and also, sometimes, common sense. I have one letter of commendation I will never forget. It was when I heard an asystole alarm in the next nursing pod on a little girl that had just arrived to the ER. When I looked in at her from the doorway I thought she was almost dead from her colour or, most likely, dying of shock. They had lost her only IV and everyone was scrambling for an IV line. She needed fluid but, more important, she needed blood products.

I had no idea why she was in the ER but it had to be bad. If they didn't get an IV in her right away she would most likely go into a cardiorespiratory arrest. She looked as white as a ghost and she had lost more blood than seemed possible and still she was alive but not for long. I reached for the IO set which was a special needle used to push or screw into a big or long bone when IVs were not able to be inserted. I never even put gloves on as they weren't in reach, and I just cleaned a spot and inserted it in a few seconds. I then hooked her IV fluid up to the IO needle and walked away. I could relax knowing the IV fluid and the blood now had a way to save her little precious body.

They now had a way to give her the lifesaving IV fluids and then administer the blood when it was ready, as she was on her way to the operating room. She would make it even if she still looked ashen. It was one time I had helped without being asked, as I wasn't willing to take a chance on losing another one. Kids can compensate for a long time and then they simply just quit and cardiac arrest is sudden but predictable if we listen to the SAMPLE history. The story of being lethargic, not crying, not eating well, with recurrent vomiting or having diarrhea for more than three days in any child is very scary. The younger they are the less reserve they will have to fight off infection and dehydration.

The younger the child, the less reserve they have and any child less than five years old who is sick is triaged as a 2 on our triage scales. Kids will get a lower number to ensure they get immediate attention. An example is a Triage of 1 is a cardiac or respiratory arrest and a Triage score of 5 is a smiling, playing kid. Sick children need to be quickly assessed, quickly treated and monitored for results or a response to our interventions and ensure we keep ahead of the illness trying to harm them.

I have seen our system kill people and I vowed to never let it happen again even if it meant losing my job. "Sometimes we will need to bend the rules to save a life but we should not break our moral code, destroy our ethics, and lose our soul along the way." This is my motto and if I lose my license or get disciplined for saving a life or standing up for anyone being lost to the system, it's fine with me.

I went back to my patients and breathed a sigh of relief but also knew I'd just made a little mistake. Currently, only our emergency doctors could perform the IO skill and I was not certified to do so as a nurse that day. I could do IOs as a paramedic and had used them before for the right reasons. I was certified at other hospitals but seeing as this was a teaching hospital the rules were also different than at the others I'd worked at in the past. Today I was bound by a different set of rules. I knew it would come up and if I got in trouble then I got in trouble. I had to do what was right morally and ethically I wasn't looking the other way.

I had a guardian angel looking after me and the little girl had me looking after her. Thank God, Darcy was in charge that day. Darcy took the hit for me and I was not going to be disciplined for helping to save a life that day. I was more than surprised to get a letter commending me for my excellent nursing skills, despite breaking a rule or two in order to save a life. I got the letter of commendation for my file. If Darcy was still my boss, I'd likely still be there getting into trouble but making the best out of every bad situation. But then it would have changed who I was and changed my life, as well, so things do happen for a reason. Everything happens for a reason and the reasons are much more complex then I will ever understand.

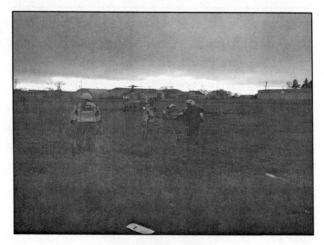

*"The Right People"*

## Chapter 25: Giving Back to the World
# "Helping Others"

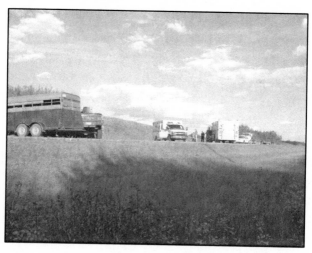

*"Giving Back—the Team"*

One of the greatest gifts I know is helping others along the paths of life. Just know not everyone has it easy and some constantly seem to be knocked down or backwards in life. I, for one, wanted to be able to help the people who needed help the most. My Grandma and Grandpa Bayliss were such amazing people in that they showed me to take people at face value and mind my own business about the rest. Grandma would say if they were bad then have nothing to do with them. Don't mention them. Don't talk bad about them, either. These were some very good lessons to learn. During the first part of my life I had nothing to offer at all but trying to help others. Eventually, I acquired the wisdom, with the ability to teach and demonstrate my medical knowledge to others, just as others had done to me over the years. I would make my living teaching others and I found my gift in helping others, especially in EMS and health care. The people we help are unmeasurable in numbers, as people then pay it forward.

The ability to share our knowledge with others is as rewarding as living somedays. Just imagine a student struggling for weeks on a skill, they struggle and struggle and one day the light clicks on and, just like that, they have it. It's a magical moment. Then imagine taking a class of twelve to twenty-four students and you have a whole page of skills to get all of them to learn and perform. One at time you start down the list of skills with each student and over time they slowly all master the skills and put the puzzle of the course together. It's so rewarding to know they have all achieved that minimum skill level and, in some cases, more. Some students will master the skill the first time and others will take longer, but in the end, they are all capable of making the grade and being successful when given a fair honest chance. Only rarely did I find a student who wasn't ever going to make the grade or had obviously chosen the wrong profession.

One time I was given a completely unexpected surprise by my own kids. My kids tried to give me a surprise airway obstruction in front of a big class of paramedic students. I went to intubate the mannequin in front of the students but the kids had put a Smartie in the airway to trick me. I tried to pass the endotracheal tube, and out of the corner of my eye I could see a surprise. I grabbed the Magill's and got it out of the way and inserted the tube. I mastered the complication and prevailed even if I was a little shocked. After they were done school I picked them up and they said "Dad, did you find our Smartie?" I gave them a scolding all while laughing. They still laugh about that little trick.

But when you have a patient gasping for breath and lying in a crowded area with all kinds of debris in the airway and poor airway positioning, bad light, and a failed laryngoscope, your day has gone to hell in a handbasket. That's why we teach students to practice until they can't get it wrong.

You will never have enough practice when everything goes wrong and that day will come sooner than later. It was common to make the students push themselves so when they had to come up with a Plan B on a failed intubation, they already had two more solutions ready to go. That is real education at its finest. That's the way students need to prepare for life. Then and only then can I take any personal credit—when I know they are ready to make the next step to be on their own as a practitioner. They can look back and think of me and the many other dedicated instructors who taught them and truly know they are ready to handle the next complicated patient.

The next greatest achievement in my life was after my personal tragedy. One dark night I was on a call in the middle of the night with my partner. We arrived at a very sick patient's residence. The family was a dynamic family looking after a senior parent, as well. It only took a few minutes and I realized we would need to bypass the patient to a city hospital and that they needed much more care then our local hospital could provide.

I called the University of Alberta Hospital and talked to the charge nurse in the ER and gave her the rundown. They were more than happy to take our patient. It helped a little as they knew me personally for years as I also still worked there as a senior nurse and as a frequent charge nurse in the busy ER. That was the easy part that night, as sometimes trying to get a patient to the most appropriate hospital was more complicated. Basically, we had to sell our story to the right agency with the right doctors and the right facility to best look after your patient. Sometimes our bypass protocols were not applicable, such as in the case of palliative care or complex patients who needed or required unique care or interventions.

While getting ready to get treatment options sorted out, we were trying to decide how to package the patient and then initiate transport all while applying initial care when my cell phone rang. That was not uncommon as we were in a poor radio area and the other crew most likely needed something. We always relied on our cell phones for a backup communication system. So, I took the call immediately while in the house I was shocked to realize it was my brother on the other end of the line. Then my world just fell apart. He said, "Dad just died." I was in the middle of a complex ALS call and I was lost as to what to do next.

I had never ever quit on a call. I was never lost for a solution to any problem or couldn't find a way out of any situation in my life time of helping others. We called Dave, the supervisor on shift, and he came to the scene right away with another EMT, Nathan, whom I have always considered one of my good friends.

We started packaging and got our patient loaded and the initial care was already done and we were ready to transport when they arrived. I explained to the family what had just happened while inside the house and they understood completely. One of the senior EMTs took over my call, and we sent it BLS as that was all we could do on short notice. Everything that we could have done ALS was already done.

I patched to the University of Alberta Hospital – Stollery and they were expecting the patient right away and would ensure care was provided as required. They also knew me and knew my world had just fallen apart. Sometimes life happens that we can't control or fix everything. If I had to finish the call I would have, but today my friends took over for me. I jumped into the back of their unit and they brought me back to base. I packed up my stuff and went home, then I took some time off and grieved for our family's loss.

It's hard to get the sad news that you lost a loved one and I had done it hundreds of times to family members over the years. Some take it very hard and some take it with no emotions. Thinking back, I called a mother one day as the ER charge nurse and told her over the phone about the loss of her son. Seeing as she wasn't in the province, I could not do anything more or in a better way as I had no idea where she even lived. She asked me to get him cremated and send his cats to the SPCA and then she just hung up on me. I thought about that a lot and still to this day can't understand how a mom could just disown her child like that. To then see a dad, punch the cement ground over and over after blaming himself for his son's death is the other side of the spectrum. I was just in shock. I didn't know what to say or what I should do.

After getting back to work I had lots of time to contemplate life, my reasons for working in EMS, and why I was teaching the courses I taught. I also wanted to know simply why I was alive and what my purpose was in this sometimes complex and unforgiving world. Out of this deep thought came the idea that I needed to make a difference. I wasn't sure of what or how this was possible. But somehow, I had to make my life count for something. I could not see myself working all my life and someday just retiring and not making a difference in this world. Life needed to have a purpose and I was going to seek a purpose for me at the same time. I just had to.

So out of the blue one day I was taking to my good friend, Norm Martineau, about my dilemma. Norm was a past student of mine and we were talking about what we could do to give back to others. Norm had also lost his dad and was working as a paramedic / LPN in the local hospital, as well as a volunteer firefighter. We came up with the idea of providing "Give Back ACLS – PALS courses" which were currently provided for registered nurses (RNs), respiratory therapists (RTs), dentists, EMT-Ps (paramedics) and doctors, primarily.

We decided it was a great idea and we set up to offer them several times a year in Tofield and in Viking, as well, when we got Kevin Formal on board. Dave Oleksyn, who was the local fire chief, as well as my partner in EMS, made it happen overnight. We borrowed equipment and, in no time, we were raising money. We contacted the Alberta Heart and Stroke Foundation and they were more than happy to participate. In no time, we had students coming from all over and trying to take our course, as it was the best. They wanted to learn in a no-stress, caring environment that had a good reputation. We made that happen out of a desire to help others and make a difference.

After three years we had raised almost $45,000 and it was all going to a great cause. We had taken all the money made from the registration which was set at $275.00 per student per course. It was all going to the Alberta Heart and Stroke Foundation to help with research into areas such as cardiac and stroke disease. We were all helping to pay it forward and giving back to others at an all-new level. After three years, I thought our "Give Back" courses were over as my employer, Lakeland College, was stopping our EMS program. It was one of the best paramedic courses in the province with some of the best instructors in the world. They were shutting it down simply for political reasons that even today are mind boggling to me, but very real just the same. Then one night I realized we weren't done yet. Up until this time we had just donated to the Heart and Stroke foundation. This was a good start but I wasn't happy at where we had just stopped. We had to come up with a way to keep the courses alive and going.

We came up with a new plan and started our fourth year of the "Give Back" courses on our own. We decided to split the money we raised among different causes. The money from the ACLS courses could support the local fire and EMS services, and the revenue from the PALS courses could go to a new group who we thought deserved and need support. We had discovered a great charity after seeing

Dr. Bill Sevcik, one of the most unique, gifted emergency physicians from the University of Alberta Hospital - Stollery, lecture on the need to help and support the Stollery Pediatric Neurosurgery Fund. We could help kids, who were a population that was very dear to us all in EMS and health care.

We wanted to help support the local fire departments and Beaver EMS, as well, this winter after we had reached our initial goal. I had set a personal goal to raise over $50,000.00 for just the Heart and Stroke Foundation and my friend Norm was right by my side all the way and he never let me down. We had a plan and we had a vision. The rest was history. So, we now had two separate goals. One was to make the $50,000.00 goal for the Heart and Stroke Foundation and the second one was to help the other groups that could use our support. There is nothing wrong with trying to reach heaven and only getting part way, as far as I am concerned. Anything is better than no attempt at all.

I told my friends I needed help again and asked them for their support one more time. Everyone was on board and they never even gave it another thought. It's such an amazing privilege to "Give Back" to our communities, to our friends, to our coworkers and to the many people out there trying to help others. It was especially good to help the thousands of our patients. The Alberta Heart and Stroke Foundation as well as our local EMS and fire departments all make this world a better place with their endless time and efforts, which are so often ignored or missed by the many people who take life for granted.

Everyone who taught the ACLS or PALS courses had seen the effect of sudden death from a cardiac arrest. We also have all seen the effects of coronary heart disease and the effects of cerebral vascular events. We all had or keep doing CPR on thousands of patients every year without even thinking about it much. It's just our job and our life dedication. We all wanted people to live without heart disease or cerebral vascular disease, which have robbed us all of family members, friends or coworkers at one time or another.

Cardiac disease and cardiac complications are the most common medical emergency in EMS and within many health care centres. We all know family members who have been robbed prematurely due to the effects of heart and stroke disease. We did cut into the private companies' attempt to make money and for that I am sorry, but we did it for the right reasons even if cost me a job or two in the long run.

We knew that our ACLS and PALS courses could help others save lives, just as teaching bystanders about using an automated external defibrillators (AEDs) that are now required by law in shopping malls, schools, arenas or at any big gathering of people does. Currently AEDs are mostly set up in the urban centres and are not as available in smaller communities, but that's changing slowly. We also strived to offer our courses to all our local EMS members, our ER and acute-care nurses, ER physicians as well as family doctors. We gave them something a little extra with each course that mattered or made a difference in our past success stories. We ensured these professionals were more than competent and ready for the complications that can and do occur regularly in prearrest or post-cardiac arrest patients.

We can all make a difference when people suffer from a cardiac event, a stroke or other circulatory-related emergency if we work as a team. We also need to promote health education and prevention to our children, teens and new adults. Finally, we need to ensure our smaller communities have the same education or access to advanced cardiac care that will ultimately then give everyone the same chance to beat the odds when suffering from a preventable disease. Rural fire departments with volunteers that provide medical response and AEDs truly shine in this area and save lives across Alberta, as well as other areas of Canada.

I could not have done any of it without Norm Martineau and Dave Oleksyn from the Tofield Fire Department, and as well as Kevin Fornal from the Viking Fire Department and Beaver EMS, and Nathan Taylor and Dan Nelson from Viking EMS. I will always be grateful to Christy Bumbac (Camrose), Cheryl Cameron (Tofield), Willy Lauder, Gary Lundman (Edmonton), and to Bob Robertson all the way from Calgary, who kept coming back to help provide and facilitate these wonderful courses to the very dedicated practitioners. Also, special thanks to many other instructors not listed who made these courses possible.

Most often the persons that we needed the most to be able to run the courses were the medical directors. The medical directors were not always on site but just a phone call away. It was our amazing medical directors who made it possible to always have medical directors available and this would typically cost from $250.00 to $500.00 per course, or up to $1400.00 if they were on-site. Right from the start I was so fortunate to get Dr. Bill Sevcik and Praveen Jain from the University of Alberta Hospital – Stollery Emergency Department to be our medical directors. For many years, they made themselves available over the phone as our medical directors at no cost. I had the privilege of working with them both for years at the University of Alberta Hospital – Stollery and they knew me well and were always there for me every time I need help. Better emergency doctors, better gentleman won't be found anywhere.

Over the years, we have had repeat student's who won't go anywhere else for courses. One of them came to one of our courses and her story made us all cry. She was working when Len and his crew and my crew picked up her daughter in cardiac arrest. We worked hard on her and Len had a pulse back before I was on scene. Then we had to deal with the stabilization, post arrest and arrange transport. We had STARS launch and we were planning on meeting them on the highway or at the closest hospital to us.

Going down the highway we had our units, police escort and fire set up a landing zone wherever we could meet. We would just pull over and close the highway off. Perform a "hot load," which means with the rotors running, and off they would go to the critical care centre in record time. You should have seen the big picture on scene as about seven staff surrounded her in the back of one ambulance and proceeded to get started on airway management, two IVs and other critical care requirements that were all happening simultaneously. There was no yelling, no speaking loudly, just team work and "Lifesaving 101" going on.

We met at the local helipad and transferred care in the back of the unit to the STARS crew and this was when my friend, the nurse, first got to see her daughter. She told us she just knew in her heart she would be okay and that she was out of the depths of dying or being lost for good. The leading ICU specialist didn't give the family much hope as when she was found in cardiac arrest and there was a time without any cerebral or brain perfusion. When someone goes into cardiac arrest, they are commonly put in an induced deep sleep to give the body and, especially, the brain time to perfuse and heal. A miracle occurred as she made it despite the downtime. In a few days, she was awake and in a few weeks, back at school. Today she is a mom and my friend is a grandma.

We will never know how many people our "Give Back" courses have touched but it's nothing short of a little miracle. I still miss my dad even when he pushed us harder than ever but I know he would approve of the result. If I knew we had helped save just one life that would be enough. I know we have done much more than that and there is much more to come from the people we helped train. I have made a difference and my friends around me have done just the same.

When we were just kids, we had an unwritten rule that we were to help our neighbours and others in times of need, no questions asked. We would drop everything and help someone and then come back and do our work or chores despite how tired or exhausted we might have been. So, that was most likely what gave us the idea for the "Give Back" programs: the loss of both our dads. Norm had a similar background to mine and anyone who knows Norm knows that as well. Working in EMS for many years as an EMT and then as a paramedic, a volunteer firefighter, and a health care worker, he had seen hell, as well.

I know Norm has his nightmares and I will always have mine. But we came by them honestly and have paid our dues despite the outcomes of life. But by helping others the nightmares and the flashbacks get a little less and that is what keeps us working and helping others. We will both just carry on until there is nothing left and that will be that. Then we will quit, but not a day before. "Quit" isn't in our vocabulary.

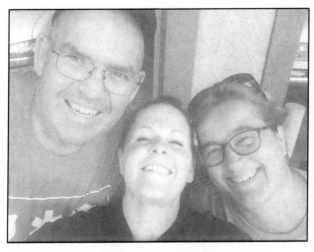

*"Walking for All of Us"*

## Chapter 26: Walking Away

# "Letting Go"

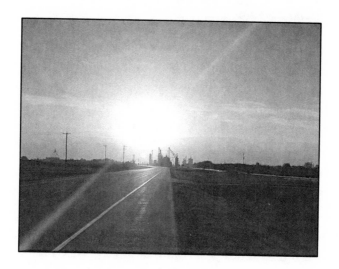

There comes a time when you need to realize that you have done what you can do and it is time to stop fighting for everyone and let others assume your role. The time is ultimately different for everyone and it comes at different times for many health care workers, I'm sure. Retirement from EMS or health care is a big step for many despite the hardships along the way with the pain and suffering that we have seen.

Essentially, we live for EMS as it's our life. Walking away or quitting means that a part of us dies as well. But in my life and for most of my life everything I did or had to do was on my terms. I was always responsible for my actions or lack of actions. I made many mistakes along the way. Surprisingly, over time I seemed to learn more and more at an alarming rate but don't really understand how or why it happened. Then one day I realized I could not and would not be able to give 110 per cent forever and regardless of how good I was today I could not wait until tomorrow to slowly give any less. I then realized I would make my own destiny on my way out, as well. Plan to walk away a few steps at a time.

Walking away is almost like calling a code too early when you have so many unanswered questions in your mind. It's like multiple internal questions from different directions are firing at your brain all at the same time and sometimes you second-guess your decisions so much you can't make any decisions at all. You can see the solutions and the right treatments but you can't get there in your current path.

It is so hard to set your radio down or not answer a pager anymore. It's almost an unconscious procedure when you get up, go to the bathroom, head outside or go downtown: you look for your radio first and your keys next and then your money last. Over the years, you either live the life of an EMS professional or you don't. I have seen many people try this industry out and decide it's not for them. There are few lifelong members in the profession. It's so sad to see the desire and need to help others but your ability to help yourself slowly takes more and more effort.

There was one event that told me it was time to leave and I do not think it was bad luck or fate just haunting my mind. The call was just like any other at the start and slowly it went in the wrong direction. Nothing would go right. The current protocols and the current thinking would not let me treat the patient the way common sense dictated. ACP, in my view, was ignoring the true needs for the EMRs and the EMTs who had missed major educational requirements in the current educational system. Many were not being given the chance to make their career fulfilling and were struggling to function as they missed the basic educational requirements right from the start of their profession. When these are missed it makes their job even harder in the real world.

We had leaders who had lost touch with reality. Some managers with our EMS services seemed to have their minds in a very dark place, some were lazy and several didn't even know what they were doing or how to manage people. Many of our managers were simply not practical or realistic. That, coupled with the fact that we were losing our battle with human life on some calls, made it very easy to reach a point of it all being too much. That was not all of it, but it was the part that broke me in the end.

One of the biggest issues is management of complex events. There comes a day when managing a call is one thing but doing a call and managing a call aren't the same. You need to be the best of the best to always give 110 percent. After seeing so many bad cases you just reach a point where you wonder why this just keep happening over and over. Drunk drivers keep killing others and never go to jail, or people keep overdosing and we just enable them. Currently we are spending millions on preventing fentanyl deaths but have never addressed the issue of why people need to take it in the first place.

Maybe I don't believe we can stop it anymore, as the whole world is spiraling downward and I don't want to go along for the ride. Pick the battles I can win and walk away from the rest is what I feel is the only way I can handle it anymore. So, when your heart isn't following along the current society trends I feel it's that much harder to manage the complex issues. The ethical and moral dilemmas along with the societal changes are hurting us all.

We need to keep from stepping on or over each other for our own personal gain. We can't bash or mentally or verbally defame others to make ourselves feel or look better to others. A few times I brought this up at work and tried to get people to realize we needed to get ready for the disaster coming, and most people ignored me saying it's not going to happen. Well, it is happening and if you think it is not you're blinded by a delusion. We are already behind the learning curve of tactical EMS. We keep ignoring the past and keep changing things for the wrong reasons. We need to be proactive and be ready for anything and everything. A disaster is only a mere minute away from all of us with no notice and no warning.

The ultimate reason to walk away now is to walk away as a winner. You need strength and endurance to fight others' battles and you can't only give 70 to 90 percent in effort. When your days are increasingly troubled with pain and decreased mobility, you realize you somehow got beaten up or worn down just too far. When you can barely walk somedays it makes you realize your best days are already gone. Over the last year, I have known pain like never before and I'm not complaining. I know I'm still alive, so that counts for everything. The pills won't help and the options for fixing a worn-out body are very limited. You don't want to show others weakness, but at the same time it's hard to concentrate when you've already exceeded your maximum limit of tolerance. It's just one more thing after another, all while just trying to look after your own needs.

So, looking ahead from looking back I think it's time to look after me now and I need to put the rest of my busy life on a shelf. I will do what it takes for me to keep going and after giving it all for so long, I want and need a rest. Time to heal me and make me physically better, spiritually better and emotionally better is my primary goal today. Matt Anderson's song "Bold and Beaten" says it best: "There's a lie behind my smile, a truth, that can't be told. It's a load that I can't share so I will carry it on my own." This is so true.

There are many things we don't and won't share with anyone. Others don't need to know our patients' or families' worst pain, or their fears with death and dying. There are too many times when during our lifetime, we see such horrific pain, the suffering and the ultimate deaths of such good people. Some who have led such a good life and don't deserve the suffering they endure in the end.

I have seen many colleagues walk away from EMS prematurely over the years and then they are lost. So, my plan to fill my days is simple. I have two golden retrievers and they are always ready and willing to go. That makes me get going, as well. The love they give me, and the bond we have, gives me a reason not to want to go to work, and slowly you lose the desire to go back to work to be beat up one more time. So why not plan to walk away and not let the system push you away? At least this way it's on my terms.

The other thing that saves me is my ability to fix or build things. I can weld, build structures, and fix lots of things, so when it comes to keeping busy I've got that covered. I may not be as gifted as my son is in wood working but I can get by so that's in my favour. I honestly think if I could afford to buy some land and farm even at a very small scale that would be the best way to walk away and just disappear. I could happily find purpose in doing my own thing and just ignore the world. As it stands now I don't watch TV. I ignore the news, hate the stupid violence on most TV shows, despise violent video games, hate politics and don't trust lawyers, which essentially makes me a redneck by most accounts, I'm sure, and that is fine with me.

I keep thinking back to the good and the bad times over my career and still have moments when I get so confused as to the why it all happened. The killing, the senseless deaths, the waste of life and the suffering that goes on and on, and people can say that's okay. From the beginning of time we have harmed others and we still have no change of heart to stop. We are the most advanced we have ever been but still we rely on gratification from seeing others hurt or lose. We see discrimination, hate and political attacks on each other in our great nation all over greed and the desire to make ourselves look better. So, in the end, I guess we all are losing the battle in life even if we think we have done so much. That would be, and has to be, the biggest reason I need to slowly just walk my own path.

I watched every episode of *NCIS* up until this year more than once and loved watching the *Longmire* series, as well. They both have lessons that make me know I'm doing the right thing or walking the right path. Gibbs is always looking after his people and no matter what, they are a family. They have each other's backs and that means so much to me. Walt from *Longmire* also is a leader and the one thing I like is that he leads even if he knows there is harm coming his way. He won't ask anyone to do what he won't do himself. But the wisdom came to me at the end of a very emotional episode of the show *The Endgame*. In it Tim McGee says so well, "Anyone can achieve their fullest potential. Who we are might be predetermined, but the path we follow is always of our choosing. We should never allow our fears or the expectations of others to set the frontiers of our destiny. Your destiny can't be changed but it can be challenged. Every man is born as many men and dies a single one." That little message says so much to me personally and, looking back on my life, I can say I followed this advice, even if I didn't realize it until right now.

No teacher in my past ever succeeded in making me feel like a loser in life. No one who tried to bully me ever won, despite making me feel bad and hurting me physically; they never made me quit. Thank God, I never gave up on life when I had no one to turn to or no place to go. Somehow, I made it, and thank God there was always someone on my side who picked me back up when I was out of options. Just when you are ready to give up, someone out of the blue comes around the corner and pulls you back on your feet.

The final part of life is just doing what I can do to help others to also succeed, even if it's on a much smaller scale. I can still help others but I want and need more time for myself and my golden retrievers need me just as much. There is no greater reward in this world than to know when you lie down at night, you have helped make the world be a little better. In years to come, the world may not miss me, but my friends will never forget me, I'm sure. That is all I can ask for; just to know my life mattered to others. We should be able to walk away from our career in peace. We should not only measure our life by our personal failures. We can clear the path for others in EMS to make their destiny a dream come true as well. After all, my EMS and health care families are the ones that count the most in the end.

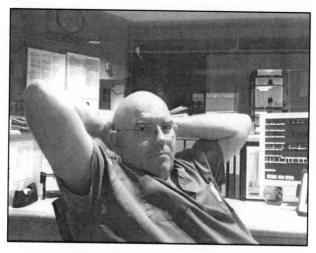

*"Thank you all for your dedication to helping others along the roads of life!" –Dale*

## Conclusions of a Lifelong Adventure

*This book is about my complex, fulfilling life in EMS, health care, medicine and the many personal events I lived through, as I can remember them. The stories and presentations are as accurate and as clear as I could portray them without hurting or harming others along the way. Along the way, I have learned so many valuable lessons. I wrote this book because I wanted to share the lessons with you all to show you a different approach to many complex and diverse situations.*

*I do not want to offend others by sharing the personal stories, the pain absorbed, as well as the misery of many all too tragic but real events. You might ask what the biggest reason to share such lifelong learning lessons and events is. Simply, I want to help to enable others to make better choices or informed decisions. Many of my past teachers and supervisors were not great role models. I hope that by sharing these stories I can help others to make better choices; after all life is too precious to waste.*

*We all need to make a difference and while working in emergency medicine, we all have a unique privilege, sadly very few will follow the pathway for a lifetime or make it their career. It should be an adventure and not just a job. I know in my heart I have made a difference in so many and have helped thousands along the way and that makes my life ever so more complete. Sadly, we have also lost all too many along the way.*

*To blame is not the solution, but by looking back and then looking forward and by sharing the lifelong lessons we have learned, we can ultimately change the future. Even by simply saving one life, we accomplish so much. By saving and helping thousands, we affect the destiny of millions around the globe. Therefore, we win no matter the sad or tragic outcomes, and the losers are the ones who refuse to change or learn from life's ongoing lessons. Admit your mistakes and keep going; never look back.*

*Thank you all for your support and for reading this somewhat painful but therapeutic account of my life. I just ask you all to pay it forward to someone in need and make this world a little better place than it was before you came along.*

*Dale M. Bayliss*

# Dedications

*I dedicate this book to the most amazing people I've had the privilege to work with throughout my career. Every one of the people listed below is precious to me and made me a better person. This book is dedicated to those who have meant so much to me, as they have enhanced my life and helped build my wonderful career of helping others.*

- *Ann Marie Baerwald, RN / EMT – Ambulance / Best Friend / Angel in Heaven*

- *Dr. Bill Sevcik / U of A – Stollery Emergency Physician / STARS / Educator*

- *Dr. Brian Rowe / U of A – Stollery / Emergency Physician / Researcher / Educator*

- *Dr. Chris Venter / Wetaskiwin Health Centre / Emergency Physician / Family Physician*

- *Dr. Christoff De Wet / Wetaskiwin Health Centre / Emergency Physician / Family Physician*

- *Dr. David Hoshizaki / U of A – ER / STARS / Emergency Physician*

- *Dr. Eddie Chang / U of A – Stollery STARS / Emergency Physician / Educator*

- *Dr. Erik Johnson / Wetaskiwin Health Centre / Emergency Physician / Family Physician*

- *Dr. Kevin Neilson / U of A – ER / STARS / Emergency Physician*

- *Dr. Layton Burkhart / U of A – ER / STARS / Emergency Physician*

- *Dr. Leanda Stassen / Wetaskiwin Health Centre / Emergency Physician / Family Physician*

- *Dr. Praveen Jain / U of A – ER / Emergency Physician / Educator*

- *Dr. Samina Ali / U of A – Stollery / Emergency Physician / Pediatrician / Researcher*

- *Dr. Simon Ward / Wetaskiwin Health Centre / Emergency Physician / Family Physician*

- *Dr. Stiaan Van Der Walt / Wetaskiwin Health Centre / Emergency Physician / Family Physician*

- *Dr. Tuhin Kumar Bakshi / Wetaskiwin Health Centre / Emergency Physician / Family Physician*

- Dr. Yunus Moolla / Wetaskiwin Health Centre / Emergency Physician / Family Physician

- Elna Eidsvik, RN / Northern Nurse / Friend for Life

- Greg Vaal / Pastor – EMT-P / My Lifesaver

- Patricia Penton / EMT-P / Lifelong EMS Friend & Coworker / Keyano EMS Program Director

**I also dedicate this book to my past coworkers at Augustana University; U of A – Augustana Campus; and Lakeland College – Camrose Campus:**

*We formed a unique team with a united front to ensure the students we taught were taught to the highest standards and that we made them the best of the best before graduation. Many of my past students would become EMS leaders as well as my future coworkers over the years and make the EMS system even better. You are all friends for life.*

- Cheryl Cameron / EMT-P / Instructor / Co-Instructor / Beaver EMS Supervisor / Coworker / Lifelong Friend

- Debbie Smeaton / Co-Director of Community Education – Manager of EMS Programs for Lakeland College / Lifelong Friend

- Heather Verbaas / EMT-P / Past Student / Co-Instructor / Beaver EMS Coworker / ACP Staff / Lifelong Friend

- Len Stelmaschuk / EMT-P / Past Student / Instructor / Co-Instructor / Camrose EMS Manager / Beaver EMS Coworker / Lifelong Friend

- Roxanne Stelmaschuk, RN / EMT-A / Augustana University;

U of A – Augustana EMS – EMR-EMT Instructor

- Tanya Blades / EMT-P / Past Student / Co-Instructor / Practicum Placements / ACP – Multiple Committee's / Lifelong Friend

- Tim Essington / EMT-P / Manager of EMS Programs / Alberta College of Paramedics (ACP) CEO / EMS Coworker / EMS Partner / Lifelong Friend

- Wes Baerg / EMT-P / Past Student / Co-Instructor / Beaver EMS Manager / Lifelong Friend

- Willy Lauder / EMT-P / Lakeland College EMS Program Instructor / ACLS - PALS - EP ACLS Instructor

**I would like to make a special dedication to the EMS family members we have lost over the course of my career: Your will always have a place in my heart for eternity.**

- *Ann Marie Baerwald, RN / EMT-A / Oxbow & Area Ambulance Service*

- *Darren Beatty / EMT-P / Wetaskiwin Emergency Medical Services / Calgary Police Service*

- *Devin Black / EMT-P / Wetaskiwin Emergency Medical Services*

- *Garry Alford / EMT-P / Alberta Health & Saskatchewan Ambulance Services Unit*

- *Lisa Glynn / EMT-P / Alberta Health Services (AHS) (Emergency Medical Services)*

- *Homer Robertson / EMT-A / Alberta Health & Saskatchewan Ambulance Services Unit*

- *Greg Turner / EMT-P /Alberta Health Services (Edmonton Emergency Medical Services)*

- *Dr. Peter Lindsay / WJ CADZOW Health Care Center – Lac La Biche / Alberta Central Air Ambulance – Physician / Alberta Heath Air Ambulance Physician / Emergency Physician / Surgeon*

**My family made it possible for me to walk down this long road:** Thanks Mum & Dad

*None of my life could have been possible without my parents. My dad, Walter S. Bayliss, was one of the hardest working men I will ever know. Dad was broken and hurt many times but never one to complain. He just got back up and kept going. Quitting was not an option. If someone needed help, my dad was there. My dad was someone who mattered.*

*My mum, Marlene A. Bayliss, raised eight kids, including two sets of twins, all within six years of each other. Mum was a rock and when we lost Dad, Mum was always there for me. She means more to me than words can ever express. As I finished the final chapter of this book, I lost my mum as well. I so wanted to show you the rewarding accomplishment.*

*This dedication to my immediate family is very important to me. My brother Donnie is my closest family member, and he and my twin sister Donna will always have me in their phone book under "Family that matters." My other family members also hold a special place in my heart even though we live so far apart.*

*Raymond and Florence Bayliss were the best grandparents in the world. (We all miss you.) You touched so many people and your dreams carry on with us. You were always there for us all as kids and we always had someplace safe and warm to go when our furnace went out. You also made the best breakfasts.*

## To the true lifesavers who matter the most to me:

| | |
|---|---|
| *Autumn Blue* | *Kevin Davison* |
| *Bill Sevcik* | *Kevin Fornal* |
| *Brent Robinson* | *Kim Showman* |
| *Brooke ter Denge* | *Len Stelmaschuk* |
| *Carla Steciuk* | *Lois Frank* |
| *Cheryl Cameron* | *Marliese Pasay* |
| *Clarrisa Turi* | *Matt Jagersma* |
| *Darlene Atkinson* | *Nathan Taylor* |
| *David Harward* | *Norm Martineau* |
| *Debbie Smeaton* | *Patricia Penton* |
| *Don & Lauren MacRae* | *Praveen Jain* |
| *Edie Chang* | *Ray Atkinson* |
| *Elna Eidsvik* | *Rena Sutherland* |
| *Erika Potvin* | *Rob Hastie* |
| *Erin Brennan* | *Rixford Smith* |
| *George Stassen* | *Samina Ali* |
| *Greg Vaal* | *Shanna Reimer* |
| *Heather Verbaas* | *Shane Loov* |
| *Joanne Meunier* | *Tanya Blades* |
| *John Anderson* | *Taylor Martz* |
| *Kelly Rairdan* | *Tim Essington* |
| *Kelmeny Laycock* | *Troy Harnish* |

And finally, to my students who carry on my legacy of caring: I can't name them all!

*"No matter where you may go, my big heart follows you."*

| | |
|---|---|
| Adriann Legate | Joe Jameson |
| Alex Jackson | John Ferris |
| Ameilia Steiger | Jon Van Sickle Kope |
| Autumn Blue | Kelly Rairdan |
| Ben Ploner | Ken Theodore |
| Belle Clark | Kent Aldous |
| Bill Johnson | Kevin Ament |
| Bob Robertson | Kevin Coaldale |
| Brent Robinson | Kevin Fornal |
| Bryce McNalley | Kevin Smyth |
| Byron Loewen | Kim Cromarty |
| Carla Steciuk | Kim Showman |
| Chantell Lynn | Len Stelmaschuk |
| Chelsea Liskiw | Linnea Mudge |
| Cheryl Cameron | Lyle Wesner |
| Clarissa Turi | Lynette Sinclair Macdonald |
| Cory Stuart | Marc Bourassa |
| Cyril Kaderabek | Marc Moebis |
| Dan Neels | Marcella Vandenberg |
| Dan Neilson | Margaret Cox |
| Dan Schmick | Mark Lowery |
| Daniel Andrew | Martin Kratochvil |
| Dave Marchand | Matt Gates |
| David Hole | Melissa Ade |
| Eleanor Maund Stephens | Melissa Grant |
| Erin Brennan | Michelle Kreinke |
| Frank Munroe | Mindy Smith |
| Glen Rea | Montana Osorio de Barros |
| Gregory Vaal | Nathan Taylor |
| Heather Blagdon | Nathan Walter |
| Heather Verbaas | Nick Mulder |
| Ian McEwan | Nick Smiley |
| Jacque Coppens | Norm Martineau |
| Jamie McCord | Pat Perkins |
| Jarrod Cohoe | Patricia Penton |
| Jeff Brausen | Pauline Wesner |
| Jeremy Rudrud | Rixford Smith |

Dale M. Bayliss

Rob Hastie
Rob Snow
Ron Oswald
Ryan O'Meara
Sam Looysen
Samuel Wolf Leg
Sara Affolder
Sarah Rae
Sasha De Vries
Seth Dodman
Shanna Reimer
Shelia Blackwood
Stacey Grant

Stephanie Donovan
Stephen Hilchie
Tammie Dale
Tanya Blades
Terry Hastings
Tim Luckwell
Tina Williams
Tony Korobanik
Tristan Donnelly
Troy Anderson
Troy Harnish
Tyler Sullivan
Tyler Vanderveen